Workbook for

Egan's Fundamentals of Respiratory Care

Eleventh Edition

Prepared By

Sandra T. Hinski, MS, RRT-NPS
Faculty, Respiratory Care Division
Gateway Community College
Phoenix, AZ

with 44 illustrations

ELSEVIER

ELSEVIER

3251 Riverport Lane
St. Louis, Missouri 63043

Notices

Previous edition copyrighted 2013, 2009, 2003, 1999

Executive Content Strategist: Sonya Seigafuse
Content Development Manager: Billie Sharp
Content Development Specialist: Heather Yocum
Publishing Services Manager: Rajendrababu Hemamalini
Senior Project Manager: Saravanan Thavamani

Printed in United States

Last digit is the print number: 9 8 7 6 5 4 3

Working together
to grow libraries in
developing countries

www.elsevier.com • www.bookaid.org

To my husband Bill and to my children Charlie and Stella, for their unwavering support and encouragement, and to all my students—past, present, and future—for providing me with the challenges that keep me learning.

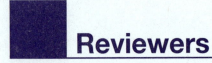

Reviewers

Greg Carter BS, RRT, AE-C
Program Director - Respiratory Program
Tacoma Community College
Tacoma, Washington

Donna Davis, BS, RRT
Director
Butte College Respiratory Care Program
Oroville, California

Contents

History of Respiratory Care

WORD WIZARD

Getting to know the terminology of medicine can be a challenge. Each chapter in this workbook starts with some word work to help you learn to "talk the talk" of a professional respiratory therapist.

Match the following terms to their definitions.

Definitions	Terms
_____ 1. Caregiver who acts as a physician extender after receiving additional education.	A. AARC
_____ 2. National professional association for respiratory care.	B. CoARC
_____ 3. Health care discipline that specializes in the promotion of optimum cardiopulmonary health.	C. NBRC
_____ 4. Name suggesting increased involvement in disease prevention and management and promotion of health and wellness.	D. cardiopulmonary system
_____ 5. One of the primary treatments for asthma uses this method of delivery.	E. respiratory care
_____ 6. Widely prescribed in hospitals by the 1940s and still a mainstay of respiratory care.	F. respiratory therapy
_____ 7. Organization responsible for the respiratory care credentialing examinations.	G. respiratory therapist(s)
_____ 8. An iron lung is an example of this therapy that helps patients who cannot breathe.	H. oxygen therapy
_____ 9. Professional organization that accredits respiratory care schools and programs.	I. aerosol medications
_____ 10. Heart and lungs working together is the "bread and butter" of our profession.	J. mechanical ventilation
_____ 11. Method to test the ways that height, age, obesity, and disease alter lung function.	K. airway management
_____ 12. Another name for the RT is this more formal term.	L. pulmonary function testing
_____ 13. Individual trained to deliver care to patients with heart and lung disease.	M. physician assistant
_____ 14. Relieving obstruction is the key to this respiratory procedure.	N. respiratory care practitioner(s)

Chapter 1 presented four main objectives for learning. Test how well you understand these mysteries of history by providing short answers to these questions.

15. Define the respiratory care profession in your own words. Include at least three main concepts. How did the profession get started? Why are we here?

16. Describe how RT schools got started. What kinds of programs do they have now? How do these programs differ from those in the early days?

SUMMARY CHECKLIST

17. Respiratory therapists apply scientific principles to _____, identify, and _____ dysfunction of the cardiopulmonary system.

18. The _____ is the professional organization for the field. It was started in _____ and was called _____.

19. The iron lung was used extensively during the _____ epidemics of the 1940s and 1950s.

FOOD FOR THOUGHT

20. Describe at least four careers that would become possible for you as a result of baccalaureate or graduate education.

    A. _____

    B. _____

    C. _____

    D. _____

21. Heroes are found in history. Name three important historical figures in respiratory care. Pick one and briefly explain how this person might inspire you in your career!

2 Delivering Evidence-Based Respiratory Care

WORD WIZARD

The Key Terms in Chapter 2 are more complicated because they describe organizations, methods for disease management, and outcome monitoring.

Increase your understanding by matching the terms below to the Big Ideas.

Term	Big Idea
1. CoARC	_____ Responsible for quality of credentialing exams
2. The Joint Commission	_____ Responsible for quality of schools
3. Evidence-based medicine	_____ Uses meta-analyses to find best care
4. NBRC	_____ Uses site visits to check quality of care

MEET THE OBJECTIVES

Fill in your answers in the spaces provided.

5. Providing quality care to the patient involves many dimensions. List three elements that are part of quality respiratory care.

    A. _____

    B. _____

    C. _____

6. Quality must be monitored to ensure it is being obtained. Give an example of each main monitoring strategy.

    A. _____

    B. _____

7. How can protocols enhance the quality of respiratory care services? Support your answer with evidence from the text.

8. Evidence-based medicine specifies precise methods for analyzing data and making decisions. Explain how this method has been used to treat ARDS. Be sure to include the ARDSNet study.

SUMMARY CHECKLIST

Complete the following statements by writing the correct term(s) in the spaces provided.

9. Ordering too many respiratory care services is called _____ and hinders delivery of quality care.

10. Specific guidelines for delivering appropriate respiratory care services are called _____.

11. The _____ respiratory therapist is the highest credential in the profession.

12. Respiratory care credentialing examinations are administered by the _____.

13. An approach to determining optimal patient management based on research is termed _____ - _____ medicine.

CASE STUDIES

Case 1

A 25-year-old woman has returned to a medical/surgical nursing unit following an appendectomy. She has no history of lung disease and is wearing a nasal cannula delivering oxygen at 3 L/min. She is alert and oriented, with a respiratory rate of 18 breaths/min and a heart rate of 82 beats/min. Her current SpO_2 (pulse oximeter reading) is 99% on the nasal cannula. Her physician orders "respiratory therapy protocol," and you are asked to assess this patient.

Use the protocol found in Figure 2-2 in the text to help you answer the following questions.

14. What are the clinical signs of hypoxia/hypoxemia? List at least three.

A. _____

B. _____

C. _____

15. Using the oxygen therapy protocol, determine if the oxygen therapy is appropriate for this patient. Support your answer with information from the textbook.

16. What action would you recommend at this time?

A 54-year-old man with a history of asthma and cigarette smoking was admitted to the hospital for a hernia repair. Following the procedure, his chest radiograph shows an elevated diaphragm and bilateral atelectasis. Vital capacity is acceptable, but the patient is unable to hold his breath. The pulse oximeter reading is 95% on room air. His heart rate is 84 beats/min, blood pressure is 110/78 mm Hg, respiratory rate is 17 breaths/min, and temperature is 36.8° C. Breath sounds are decreased bilaterally with apical wheezes. He has a weak nonproductive cough. The patient is alert and oriented.

17. Use the algorithm in Figure 2-1 in the text to determine how to give this patient his medications. If you've never used an algorithm before, it may be useful to write out the steps in your path. Start with "Is the patient alert?" and write your answer in Step 1.

Step 1 _____

Step 2 _____

Step 3 _____

Step 4 _____

WHAT DOES THE NBRC SAY?

Circle the best answer for the following multiple choice questions.

18. A patient with chronic obstructive pulmonary disease complains of difficulty breathing when he is ambulating. His SpO_2 is 88% at rest. Which of the following would you recommend?
    A. Oxygen therapy
    B. PEEP therapy
    C. Antibiotic therapy
    D. Aerosolized bronchodilator therapy

19. An alert 18-year-old patient is admitted with difficulty breathing. The patient receives a diagnosis of asthma, and you are asked to instruct the patient in the use of an MDI. An MDI is a device used for
    A. oxygen therapy.
    B. PEEP therapy.
    C. antibiotic therapy.
    D. aerosolized bronchodilator therapy.

20. A patient with pneumonia is receiving oxygen via nasal cannula at 2 L/min. The SpO_2 is 89%, heart rate is 110 beats/min, and respiratory rate is 24 breaths/min. Which of the following would you recommend?
    A. Increase the liter per minute flow to the cannula.
    B. Intubate and begin mechanical ventilation.
    C. Initiate aerosolized bronchodilator therapy.
    D. Initiate postural drainage.

21. Protocol-based therapy and quality assurance efforts do not always work! Discuss some of the reasons you think these two strategies might fail.

22. Evidence-based medicine (EBM) uses meta-analysis. What does this term mean? Why is meta-analysis different from standard reviews of literature? Is it better?

Chapter **2** **Delivering Evidence-Based Respiratory Care**

3 Quality, Patient Safety, and Communication, and Recordkeeping

WORD WIZARD

Read Chapter 3 in your textbook and see if you can fill in the missing words.

Health care settings are filled with electrical equipment. The flow of electricity is called _____. Everything should have a three-prong plug. The third prong is the neutral wire, or _____, which helps prevent electrocution. For this reason, no outside electrical devices are allowed in the hospital unless the biomedical staff checks them. Electrocution can occur in the form of a(n) _____ shock. This might happen if you are standing on a wet floor and a power cord falls onto the floor. Many power cords are detachable, so this is a potential hazard. Always clean up spills.

A small shock, or _____ shock, is a hazard to patients who have pacemakers, ECG leads, and indwelling heart catheters. These shocks may result in ventricular fibrillation and death! This could happen if the _____ wire gets broken, so don't ever roll beds or other equipment over electrical power cords. Report frayed cords and take suspect equipment out of use.

Because high oxygen concentrations are used in respiratory care, fire is a real hazard.

Even though oxygen is categorized as a(n) _____ gas and does not burn, it greatly speeds up an existing fire.

In fact, oxygen is necessary for fires to exist. For a fire to start, you also need _____, material, and heat.

Remove any of these three, and the fire will go out. You must make sure that ignition sources such as _____ are not allowed when oxygen is in use. Most hospitals will call a "Code Red" if a fire exists, and you must respond. One of the respiratory therapist's responsibilities in a fire is to shut off the zone valve to the affected area if the fire is near a patient using oxygen. (See Chapter 40, Storage and Delivery of Medical Gases.)

KEEP IT MOVING!

The following are some guidelines for safe ambulation. Number them 1 through 7 in the right order.

_____ Dangle the patient.

_____ Sit the patient up.

_____ Assist to a standing position.

_____ Encourage slow, easy breathing.

_____ Lower the bed and lock the wheels.

_____ Move the IV pole close to the patient.

_____ Provide support while walking.

Fill in your answers in the spaces provided.

1. List three risks that are common among patients receiving respiratory care.

   A. _____

   B. _____

   C. _____

2. Describe two problems associated with immobility and two benefits of ambulation.

   A. _____

   B. _____

3. What is the main reason you should use good body mechanics?

4. List two factors you should monitor during patient ambulation. (There is a total of five!)

   A. _____

   B. _____

5. List four factors that influence the communication process.

   A. _____

   B. _____

   C. _____

   D. _____

6. The text lists five ways to improve your effectiveness as a sender of messages. Describe two of these that apply to you. Give examples of situations where you communicated well (or not!).
   I need to improve in...

   A. _____

   B. _____

   Give an example of good communication.

   Give an example of bad communication.

7. Name four sources of conflict in health care organizations. Give an example of each.

A. _____

B. _____

C. _____

D. _____

8. What is a medical record? Who owns the record? Who is allowed to read it?

9. State one legal and one practical essential aspect of recordkeeping.

A. _____

B. _____

10. One of the most common formats that respiratory therapists (and others) use in charting is the SOAP format. What does SOAP mean? Give examples of information you would chart for each category.

	MEANING	EXAMPLE
S		
O		
A		
P		

SUMMARY CHECKLIST

Complete the following statements by writing the correct term(s) in the spaces provided.

11. You should begin _____ as soon as a patient is stable.

12. A(n) _____ is a small current that enters the body through external catheters and may cause ventricular fibrillation.

13. Prevent electrical shocks by always _____ your equipment.

14. You can minimize fire hazards by removing flammable materials and ignition sources from areas where _____ is in use.

15. _____ skills play a key role in your ability to achieve desired patient outcomes.

16. Accommodating, avoiding, collaborating, competing, and compromising are basic strategies for handling _____.

17. A medical record is a _____ document.

18. You must _____ each treatment, medication, or procedure you provide.

Chapter **3** Quality, Patient Safety, and Communication, and Recordkeeping

Case 1

The physician orders ambulation for a patient who is receiving oxygen. The nurse asks you to assist. The patient is in bed wearing a nasal cannula running at 2 L/min.

19. What equipment will you need *before* you try to walk with this patient?

After 5 minutes of walking, you notice that the patient is breathing at a rate of 24 breaths/min and using his accessory muscles of ventilation. His skin appears sweaty, and he is exhaling through pursed lips.

20. What observations are important to note in this situation? What action would you take?

Case 2

You are caring for a patient who is on a mechanical ventilator. You need to transport the patient to radiology for a CT scan. The nurse unplugs the IV pump and pulse oximeter from the *back* of each unit. The pumps and the pulse oximeter are now running on their battery systems. As you prepare to leave, you notice that the power cords are still plugged into the wall outlets. The physician and the nurse are anxious to get the transport under way.

21. Describe the actions you would take if you encountered this situation.

22. What potential conflict/communication problems exist? How would you deal with them?

Circle the best answer for the following multiple choice questions.

23. A respiratory therapist has completed SOAP charting in the progress notes following a bronchodilator treatment. While signing the chart form, she notices that the wrong amount for the medication has been entered. Which of the following actions should be done at this time?
    1. Draw one line through the error.
    2. Notify the physician of the error.
    3. Write "Error" and initial.
    4. Recopy the progress notes.
        A. 1 and 2
        B. 1 and 3
        C. 2 and 4
        D. 3 and 4

24. A patient with asthma has orders for albuterol by medication nebulizer every 2 hours. During the shift, the patient improves, and the order is changed to every 4 hours. In regard to the new frequency, what action should you take?
    1. Note the change in your charting.
    2. Inform the registered nurse of the order.
    3. Frequency will change during your shift.
        A. 1 and 2
        B. 1 and 3
        C. 2 and 3
        D. 1, 2, and 3

25. A patient's heart rate increases from 88 to 134 beats/min following a breathing treatment. After reassuring the patient, the respiratory therapist should
    A. discontinue the therapy.
    B. reduce the dosage of the medication.
    C. place the patient on oxygen.
    D. notify the physician.

FOOD FOR THOUGHT

26. What do you think is the most common type of injury in health care?

27. On what shift do most injuries, accidents, and patient incidents occur?

28. Explain the Plan-Do Study-Act cycle.

4 Principles of Infection Prevention and Control

Match the key definition with the correct term.

Definitions	Terms
_____ Infections that are acquired in the hospital.	A. Fomites
_____ Inanimate objects that help transfer pathogens.	B. Nosocomial
_____ Death of all microorganisms.	C. Sterilization
_____ Universal method of protection for health workers.	D. Disinfection
_____ Death of pathogenic microorganisms.	E. Standard precautions

MEET THE OBJECTIVES

Fill in your answers in the spaces provided.

1. What is a health care–associated infection (HAI)? How many people develop this type of infection?

   A. HAI = _____

   B. How many people develop this type of infection? _____ What percentage of patients is this?

   _____

2. Why is knowledge regarding HAIs important to our profession?

3. List three elements that are required for these infections to develop.

   A. _____

   B. _____

   C. _____

4. A susceptible host may be elderly, have HIV, or be undergoing chemotherapy, but we can still reduce host susceptibility by focusing on employee health and chemoprophylaxis. List five vaccinations that might help you decrease the risk of transmitting an HAI.

A. _____

B. _____

C. _____

D. _____

E. _____

5. Respiratory therapists must know the routes of disease transmission so we can avoid infection. What are the three **major** routes? Give an example of each.

	ROUTE	EXAMPLE
A.		
B.		
C.		

6. Define the following equipment processing definitions.

TERM	DEFINITION
Cleaning	
Disinfection (general term)	
Disinfection, low-level	
Disinfection, intermediate-level	
Disinfection, high-level	
Sterilization	

7. You will need to decide how to clean the RT equipment. Use the Mini-Clini on "Selection of Equipment Processing Methods" of your text to help decide how to disinfect and sterilize these items:

ITEM	DISINFECT	STERILIZE
A. Laryngoscope blade		
B. Humidifier		
C. Mechanical ventilator		

8. List the three general barrier methods to prevent exposure to organisms. Describe a situation or identify an organism for which you (as a respiratory therapist) would need this type of protection.

A. _____

B. _____

C. _____

Complete the following statements by writing the correct term(s) in the spaces provided.

9. _____ is the best choice for high-level disinfection of semicritical respiratory care equipment.

10. Among respiratory care equipment, _____ have the greatest potential to spread infection.

11. Always use _____ fluids for tracheal suctioning and filling nebulizers and humidifiers.

12. Wear _____ and _____ during any procedure that can generate splashes or sprays of body fluids.

13. The use of _____ is part of routine care when there is skin contact.

14. The maximum duration of time that ventilator circuits can be used safely is _____.

CASE STUDIES

Case 1

You work in the surgical intensive care unit (ICU) of a large urban hospital. Over the past 2 days, a number of patients in the unit have developed serious *Staphylococcus aureus* infections.

15. Why do postoperative patients have an increased risk of infection?

16. What is the most common source of *S. aureus* organisms?

17. Identify three ways to disrupt the route of transmission in this situation.

    A. _____

    B. _____

    C. _____

Case 2

During the third day of your clinical rotation, you are assigned to a therapist who has an extremely heavy workload on a medical floor of the hospital. The therapist puts on gloves for each patient contact and asks you to do so also. When you go to wash your hands after the first treatment, the therapist tells you, "We don't have time for that, and besides the gloves will keep our hands clean."

18. Explain the role of gloves in protecting practitioners and preventing the spread of infection.

19. What does the CDC say about cleaning your hands in regard to washing? Are there any alternatives?

Case 3

A serious tuberculosis outbreak occurs in a local prison facility. You are called to the emergency department as four of the sickest patients are being admitted together to your hospital for treatment.

20. By what route does tuberculosis spread?

21. When transporting these patients out of the emergency department, what action should you take?

22. What kinds of precautions should be taken to prevent the spread of infection once these patients are admitted?

23. What special guidelines exist in regard to cough-inducing and aerosol-generating procedures for patients with active tuberculosis?

24. What other concerns do you have in working with these patients?

25. What should you do if enough private rooms with airborne precautions are not available for this group of patients?

WHAT DOES THE NBRC SAY?

Circle the best answer for the following multiple choice questions.

The following questions refer to this situation:

A 72-year-old female patient with COPD has a tracheostomy tube in place following prolonged intubation and mechanical ventilation. She is currently in the medical intensive care unit. After you take her off the ventilator, you will need to set up a heated aerosol system with an FiO_2 of 40%.

26. What type of water should be placed in the nebulizer?
    A. Distilled water
    B. Tap water
    C. Normal saline solution
    D. Sterile distilled water

27. To help lower the risk of a nosocomial infection when using heated aerosol systems, the respiratory therapist should do which of the following?
    1. Label the equipment with the date and time it is started.
    2. Avoid draining the tubing to prevent contamination.
    3. Use aseptic technique during the initial setup.
    4. Use a filter or heat and moisture exchanger (HME) to reduce airborne bacteria.
        A. 1 and 3
        B. 1 and 2
        C. 2 and 4
        D. 3 and 4

28. The best way to prevent the spread of infection in the ICU is to
    A. ensure that sterilized equipment is used.
    B. wash your hands after every patient contact.
    C. wear gloves when you come in contact with body fluids.
    D. isolate infected patients.

29. One of your fellow students comes to clinical rotation with a cold. He asks you not to tell your clinical instructor because missed clinical days are hard to make up. What is your reaction to this situation? What are the potential problems with this scenario?

30. The college recommends that you get immunized against hepatitis B before attending clinical rotation. The consent form lists a number of possible side effects of the vaccine, and the vaccination is expensive. What are the pros and cons of vaccines? What will you choose?

5 Ethical and Legal Implications of Practice

WORD WIZARD

Complete the following paragraph by writing the correct terms in the spaces provided.

The two basic types of law in the United States are public law and civil law. Public law is further divided into

administrative law and _____ law. Health care facilities operate under a mountain of regulations set by

government agencies. Private, or _____, law protects citizens who feel they have been harmed. The individual

who brings a complaint is called the _____, and those accused of wrongdoing are known as _____.

A(n) _____ is a civil wrong. These cases could easily involve a health care practitioner. There are three types

of civil law cases. _____ is the failure to perform your duties competently. Cases in which the patient falls,
is given the wrong medication, or is harmed by equipment revolve around a provider's duty to anticipate harm and
prevent it from happening.

Expert testimony, professional guidelines, or even circumstantial evidence can determine what a reasonable and pru-

dent respiratory therapist would have done in a given situation. The Latin term _____ ("the thing speaks for
itself") is sometimes invoked to show that harm occurred because of inappropriate care. When a professional fails to act

skillfully, breaches ethics, or performs below a reasonable standard, it is called _____. Wrongdoing may be

considered intentional or unintentional. Intentional acts include _____, or placing another person in fear of

bodily harm, and _____, or physical contact without consent. Other common intentional harm occurs through

_____, which is verbal defamation of character, and _____, which is written defamation of char-

acter. Finally, information about patients is considered private, or _____, and cannot be shared with anyone
who is not involved in their care.

MEET THE OBJECTIVES

1. The basis of ethics is found in philosophy and is a science in itself. What is the fundamental question of ethics?

2. What is the one primary purpose of a professional code of ethics?

3. Describe some of the information you might gather or consider before making a decision that involves ethics. For example, before discontinuing life support for a patient who is brain dead, what might you consider?

4. Health care is constantly changing and evolving in ways that affect ethical and legal decision making. Please discuss one example, such as managed care, and briefly explain how this new kind of medicine might shape our choices.

CASE STUDIES

Case 1

You get a chance to meet with your fellow students for lunch in the hospital cafeteria during a busy clinical day. One of your classmates is bursting with excitement as you sit down to eat. "You won't believe what I got to do today! I was taking care of Mr. Brainola, a patient in the intensive care unit (ICU), and he started to go bad, and we had to intubate. Then he coded, and I got to do CPR! It was so cool!"

5. What's the problem with this picture? What violation has your classmate committed?

6. What are the possible consequences of this scenario?

7. What action should you take?

8. Is this situation simply a breach of ethics or a violation of law?

19

You receive an order to administer a bronchodilator to a 27-year-old asthma patient. The patient refuses the therapy, stating, "I just can't take any more of this today!" He appears alert and oriented.

9. Does the patient have a legal right to refuse in this case? Cite evidence from the text to justify your answer.

10. How would you respond to this situation?

11. What other action should you take at this time?

After finishing with the previous patient, you receive a stat call to the orthopedic floor. The registered nurse informs you they are having problems with a 76-year-old woman who recently had surgical repair of a broken hip. As you enter the room, you notice that she has removed her oxygen mask. She is breathing rapidly, and her color is not good. The pulse oximeter shows a saturation of 84%. When you try to get the patient to wear the oxygen mask, she screams at you to get out of the room.

12. Does the patient have a legal right to refuse in this case? Cite evidence from the text to justify your answer.

13. How would you respond to this situation?

Chapter **5** **Ethical and Legal Implications of Practice**

14. Would physical restraints be an option or a possible case of battery?

CASE STUDIES

Case 1

A 17-year-old male is admitted for pneumonia. This young man is depressed and has expressed thoughts of ending his life if "my worst fears are true about this illness." Laboratory studies reveal that the patient is HIV positive. His physician expresses concern to the other caregivers about revealing the patient's diagnosis to him.

15. Under what circumstances can you lie (or not tell the truth) to patients?

16. What are your feelings about telling the truth to patients?

17. What would you do if the patient asks you if he has AIDS?

Ethical Decision-Making Model

Let's apply the ethical decision-making model to Case 1 (see Box 5-2 in your text). Write your answers in the spaces provided.

18. What is the problem or issue in this case?

19. Who are the individuals involved?

20. What ethical principle(s) apply here?

21. Who should make the decision to tell the patient?

22. What is your role as a respiratory therapist who is giving treatments to this patient?

23. Are there short-term consequences to either decision? Long-term consequences?

24. Make the decision! (What would you do?)

25. How would you proceed after you made your choice?

A respiratory therapist who is a deeply religious individual has strong feelings about homosexuality. When he is assigned to provide therapy for an openly homosexual patient, he objects to the supervisor, saying, "I do not want to take care of him. It is against my religious principles. Assign someone else."

26. What are some of the possible problems for the respiratory department that could arise out of this situation?

27. Patients are allowed to refuse even life-sustaining treatment for religious reasons. What about professional caregivers?

28. What would you do if you were the supervisor?

SUMMARY CHECKLIST

Complete the following statements by writing the correct terms in the spaces provided.

29. The two basic ethical theories are _____ and _____.

30. _____ deals with the relationships of private parties and the government.

31. Professional _____ is negligence in which a professional has failed to provide the _____ expected, resulting in _____ to someone.

32. Practitioners must carry out their duties with an eye toward _____ themselves in the case of _____ action.

33. A(n) _____ act defines who can perform specified duties in health care. The purpose of _____ is to provide for the public's safety.

34. You are asked to do a clinical case study by your instructor. What is PHI? What information do you think you should remove from the case to avoid identifying the patient to others?

35. What is the difference between an advance directive and a living will?

6 Physical Principles of Respiratory Care

WORD WIZARD

Complete the following paragraph by writing the correct terms in the spaces provided.

Without humidity, our airways get irritated and mucus gets thick and difficult to expectorate. The actual amount, or weight, of water vapor in a gas is called _____ humidity. As respiratory therapists, we compare the weight of water vapor to the amount it could hold if the gas were fully saturated. This ratio of content to capacity is known as _____ humidity. You hear about this on the weather report every day. I'm more interested in how much vapor gas can hold inside the airways. This amount is called percent _____ humidity. When inspired gas has less than 100% of its capacity, a humidity _____ exists. Humidifiers are used to make up the difference. When you get a can of cold soda on a hot day, water droplets begin to form on the outside of the can. That's because the air around the can is cooling (cold air does not hold as much water vapor as warm air). When air cools and gaseous water returns to a liquid form, we say that _____ has occurred. The opposite effect occurs when the drink warms. Water molecules escape from the liquid into the air. This process is called _____ and adds to the humidity in the air.

Heat moves in mysterious ways—four of them, to be precise. Newborn babies are especially sensitive to heat loss. Keeping a preemie warm can make the difference between life and death! When babies are born, we dry them off to prevent loss through _____. Then they are wrapped in cloth to prevent _____, or loss that occurs from contact with a cooler object. Finally, we may put them in incubators. The incubator provides warmth in two ways. First, a special light _____ heat toward the baby. Second, warm air blows into the incubator. Transfer of heat through movement of fluids (or gas) is called _____.

MEET THE OBJECTIVES

1. Oxygen normally exists as a gas at sea level. What has to happen to turn gaseous oxygen into liquid oxygen for medical use?

2. What happens to the temperature when liquid oxygen is converted into gaseous oxygen?

3. Describe the two major types of internal energy. Which form is most likely the cause of the internal energy of gases?

4. At sea level, what is the primary factor that determines the state of matter?

5. Liquid water can easily turn into its gaseous or vapor form. Water vapor content of gas is important for comfort and airway health. What factors affect the amount and rate of vaporization of water?

6. Explain why visible moisture, a mist, appears when you exhale on a cold day.

7. What is the name of the primary law that governs resistance, or opposition, to flow through the airway and the amount of pressure, or work, that must be performed to overcome resistance and move air in and out?

OBEY THE LAWS

This section provides some real examples of gas laws in action.

In the spaces provided, identify which law is being demonstrated.

Example 1
A registered pulmonary function technologist (RPFT) is performing lung testing on a patient. The patient inhales 1.5 L from the spirometer.

8. What will happen to the volume of gas inside the patient's lungs?

9. What is the gas law?

Example 2
A home care respiratory therapist places an oxygen cylinder in a van so that she can take it to a client's house. The van catches on fire.

10. What will happen to the pressure inside the cylinder as it gets warmer?

11. What is the gas law?

Example 3

When you start to inhale, your diaphragm drops and your chest expands. In other words, you increase the size, or volume, of your chest.

12. What happens to the pressure inside your chest?

13. What is the gas law?

TRY IT, YOU'LL LIKE IT!

Here are some safe, easy experiments you can perform in the laboratory at school or at home.

Experiment 1

Place a dry, empty *glass* soda bottle in the freezer for at least 15 minutes. Take the bottle out and *immediately* cover the mouth of the bottle with a balloon. Wait a few minutes and watch!

14. What happened to the balloon?

15. Which gas law is responsible for the result?

Experiment 2

Cut out a 1-inch-wide strip of notebook paper. Hold one end of the paper to your chin, just below your lip. Blow steadily across the top of the paper.

16. What happened to the paper?

17. What principle is responsible for this action?

Another experiment that shows this same principle can be accomplished with balloons. Blow up two round balloons and tie them off. Attach about 1 foot of string to each balloon. Tape the string to a stick (such as a ruler or yardstick) so the balloons are about 6 to 8 inches apart. Blow between the balloons.

18. What happened to the balloons?

Experiment 3

Get a coffee stirrer, an ordinary straw, and a big straw (like the kind you use for a milkshake). Now get two cups. Put some water in one cup. Put some honey in another. Suck the water up through each straw. Now try the honey. To make this more interesting, get a 6-foot length of oxygen-connecting tubing. Try the two fluids again!

19. Which tube is easiest to suck through?

20. Which fluid is easiest to suck up?

21. Which gas law explains all this?

Experiment 4

Surface tension can be a hard concept to grasp, but it is easy to demonstrate. Take a cup or glass and fill it with water up to the top. Slowly add more water until the cup is about to overflow. Observe the water surface as it sits slightly above the rim of the cup.

22. Which gas law explains your ability to fill a cup above the rim without its overflowing?

23. What is the name of the curved surface of the water?

CASE STUDIES

Case 1

A respiratory therapist decides to attend the AARC International Congress. To get there, the therapist must travel by air. Before taking off, the flight attendant explains the oxygen system. The therapist pays attention when he sees the partial rebreathing mask. He also knows that something interesting happens to oxygenation at 30,000 feet.

24. What is the barometric pressure (P_B) and partial pressure of inspired oxygen (PiO_2) at this altitude?

P_B _____

PiO_2 _____

25. A properly fitting oxygen mask can deliver about 70% oxygen to passengers. What would the PiO_2 be while wearing the mask?

26. Which gas law did you use to make these conclusions?

Case 2

Respiratory therapists frequently draw arterial blood samples to measure the partial pressures of oxygen and carbon dioxide in the blood. Many patients have elevated or decreased body temperatures.

27. What effect does a fever have on these partial pressure readings?

28. A normal arterial carbon dioxide pressure (PaCO₂) is 40 mm Hg (torr) at a body temperature of 37° C. Estimate the new PaCO₂ if body temperature is 40° C.

29. Why is temperature correction of arterial blood gas readings controversial?

MATHEMATICS

30. Convert 30° C to degrees Kelvin.

Formula _____

Solution _____

Answer _____

31. Convert 68° F to degrees Celsius.

Formula _____

Solution _____

Answer _____

32. Convert 40° C to degrees Fahrenheit.

Formula _____

Solution _____

Answer _____

33. At body temperature, gas has a saturated capacity of about 44 mg of water vapor per liter. If a gas has an absolute humidity of 22 mg/L, what is the relative humidity?

Formula _____

Solution _____

Answer _____

34. What is the humidity deficit in Question 33?

Formula _____

Solution _____

Answer _____

35. Convert a pressure reading of 10 millimeters of mercury (mm Hg) to centimeters of water (cm H₂O).

Formula _____

Solution _____

Answer _____

Chapter **6** **Physical Principles of Respiratory Care**

36. Convert a pressure reading of 10 centimeters of water (cm H_2O) to kilopascals (kPa). Hint: It's okay to round off.

Formula _____

Solution _____

Answer _____

37. Air is normally about 21% oxygen. Calculate the partial pressure of oxygen in air (PiO_2) when the barometric pressure is 760 mm Hg.

Formula _____

Solution _____

Answer _____

38. Now calculate the new PiO_2 that would result if the barometric pressure is 500 mm Hg.

Formula _____

Solution _____

Answer _____

SUMMARY CHECKLIST

39. Two temperature scales are used in hospitals in the United States. The _____ scale is used universally in health care around the world.

40. Transfer of heat energy can occur through _____, convection, radiation, and _____.

41. The total _____ pressure of a mixture of gases must equal the sum of the _____ pressures of the constituent gases.

42. A gas's _____ and pressure vary directly with _____.

43. When temperature is constant, a gas's volume and pressure vary _____.

WHAT DOES THE NBRC SAY?

44. A blood gas analyzer is being calibrated with a 5% mixture of carbon dioxide and balance nitrogen. If the barometric pressure is 747 mm Hg, what reading would be most correct for the CO_2 electrode of the analyzer?
    A. 35 mm Hg
    B. 37 mm Hg
    C. 7.47 mm Hg
    D. 74.7 mm Hg

45. What is the most significant factor affecting airway resistance?
    A. Airway length
    B. Airway radius
    C. Gas viscosity
    D. Gas flow rate

FOOD FOR THOUGHT

46. What property of liquid oxygen makes it especially difficult and potentially harmful to work with at home?

Chapter **6** **Physical Principles of Respiratory Care**

7 E-Medicine in Respiratory Care

WORD WIZARD

Complete the following paragraph by writing the correct term in the blank provided.

Talk to Me!

Computers can talk to each other through local networks inside the hospital or networks outside the institution. The global network of computer networks is called _____. Inside the hospital, a similar network called the _____ serves as a conduit for information. The term that relates to the use of computerized or digital technology to enhance efficiency and effectiveness of health care in general and more specifically patient care is called _____. _____ refers to the use of information technology in health care and combines advances in computer science and technology to improve clinical care, manage the health of populations, and accelerate research.

COMPUTERS IN HEALTH CARE

Clinicians use computers to help interpret data, reach a diagnosis, and automate certain aspects of patient care. Fill in your answers in the spaces provided.

1. What do EHR and EMR stand for? Define and explain the difference between the two.

   A. EHR: _____

   B. EMR: _____

   Define and explain: _____

   _____

   _____

2. What is a PACS and how does it help respiratory therapists in the critical care setting?

3. What are the advantages of wireless handheld systems? List three.

   A. _____

   B. _____

   C. _____

4. What does the term "benchmarking" mean? How does a manager use benchmarking to assess performance?

5. Health care providers are using computers in the area of disease prevention. Tell us a little more about the following two applications of information technology. How will respiratory therapists use technology to better care for patients?

   A. Tobacco cessation: _____

   _____

   _____

   B. Disease management: _____

   _____

   _____

6. What is telemedicine?

7. What is VBP and what agency implemented it?

CASE STUDY

Case 1

A respiratory care student is asked by her instructor to explain how to tell if information from a website is likely to be trustworthy. While reading Chapter 7, the student learned about a code of conduct for medical and health websites that would provide the information she needed. What term indicates that a website shows clearly the source of information and the date when the page was modified?

_____

8. Justifiability is a critical concept in evaluating claims that a product, device, or drug will benefit patients. Explain this concept and why it is important.

9. Explain the phrase "transparency of sponsorship."

10. What difference do ads make?

Activity 1: Respiratory Care

In this exercise, you will locate a specific document from the AARC's website.
- Open the AARC home page (www.aarc.org).
- Click on "Resources" and find the section on Clinical Practice Guidelines (CPGs).
- Open the guideline on pulse oximetry.
- Print this guideline and use it as a study reference. Why? One reason is the reliability of this material. Another good reason is that the National Board for Respiratory Care says in its newsletter, "CPGs are a valuable tool for preparing for board examinations."

  How about that! The AARC website is the single most useful resource for respiratory therapy students and practitioners on the internet.

FOOD FOR THOUGHT

It is easy to learn how to use the computer for more than just games. Aside from the activities listed earlier, you may want to try the following:
- Locate the home page for your college.
- If your program of study has a website, locate it and print the home page or find some specific information from the page. If you do not have a page, find one from another program. These sites are easily accessed from the AARC website.
- If you do not have a program website, design one as a class project. Ask your media or learning center to provide skills and access to the campus server. With the software now available, it is easy to learn to make a website.

A FINAL THOUGHT

Smartphones, iPods, and other handheld devices can be invaluable. There are many very useful medical applications for these devices, and many are free to download. For example, there is a program that allows users to look up almost any drug and check dosages, costs, side effects, and so on. Also available is a blood gas calculator, Henderson-Hasselbalch calculator, peak flow and PFT norms, cylinder duration—you name it. Many students buy handheld devices because there is no better digital tool. You can shoot video of procedures in the laboratory or take photos of equipment for study purposes. Plus they fit in your lab coat pocket! (But remember, don't take pictures in the hospital.)

8 Fundamentals of Respiratory Care Research

1. Fill in the definitions of the following key words.

	KEY WORD	DEFINITION
A.	Bibliographic database	
B.	PubMed	
C.	Portals	
D.	Synthesized database	
E.	Hypothesis	
F.	Research protocols	

HOW TO BE A SCIENTIST

2. List in order the outline a research paper typically follows.

   A. _____

   B. _____

   C. _____

   D. _____

   E. _____

3. Which section of a research paper explains what was done to answer the research question?

4. What does IRB stand for?

5. What are *peer reviewers* and what is their purpose regarding research papers?

6. What three outcome recommendations can a peer reviewers give to the journal editor about the submitted research paper?

A. _____

B. _____

C. _____

7. Try to develop a study idea. Choose and define a research topic area and write it down. _____

8. Go to the library website of your educational institution and use a bibliographic database to research your idea. Attempt the following activity.

A. Go to the following website: http://www.ncbi.nlm.nih.gov/pubmed

B. Enter one key word in the first search field and click search. (Make sure the box to the left of the search field has PubMed displayed.) How many results did you get? _____

C. Using the tab on the left column, limit your results to those published in the last 5 years. How many results did you get? _____

D. What is one way you can narrow your search? _____

E. Now, add an additional key word to your initial key word in the search field using the word "AND" to separate the words. How many results did you get? (Hint…look up what a Boolean operator is.) _____

F. Under the search field click on the "Advanced" link. What happens? _____

G. What is a MeSH term and how is it used? _____

H. Clear your original search field. Now, go to the box to the left of the search field that currently has "PubMed" displayed and change it to "MeSH" in the search field.

I. Now begin to type your original key word. What happened? _____

J. Find an article, open it, and evaluate the sources using the following categories.
   i. Relevance
      1. Does the information relate to your topic or question?
      2. What is the intended audience?
   ii. Currency
      1. When was the article published?
   iii. Authority (Remember, scholarly articles are written by experts and reviewed by experts!)
      1. What are the author's credentials or organizational affiliations?
      2. Is the research sponsored by a particular organization/company/agency?
   iv. Accuracy
      1. Is the information supported by evidence?
      2. Are there any spelling or grammatical errors?
   v. Purpose
      1. What is the purpose of the information? To inform? Teach? Sell a product? Persuade?
      2. Are there any political, ideological, institutional, or personal biases?
      3. Does the point of view appear to be objective and impartial?

K. Does your educational institution have any expert tools to aid in creating citations? What is a common citation format for peer-reviewed articles? (Hint: Make an appointment with a librarian for help. They are a great resource!)

9 The Respiratory System

WORD WIZARD

Fill in the box below regarding medical terminology.

	MEDICAL TERMINOLOGY	IN PLAIN LANGUAGE, PLEASE
A.	Alveoli	Tiny air sacs for gas exchange
B.		Place where trachea splits into R+L
C.	Cilia	
D.		Primary muscle of breathing
E.	Epiglottis	
F.		Hole that opens into your windpipe
G.	Hilum	
H.		Voice box
I.	Pharynx	
J.		Wrapping that lines the lungs
K.	Sternum	
L.		Windpipe

FETAL FACTS

1. During what stage and week of development is alveolar capillary surface area considered sufficient to support extrauterine life?

   Stage: _____

   Week: _____

2. What is the primary organ of gas exchange for the fetus?

3. Describe the umbilical cord blood vessels.

4. The fetus lives in a relatively hypoxic environment. What is considered to be a major factor that enables the fetus to survive under these conditions?

5. About half of the blood entering the right atrium is shunted to the left atrium via what structure?

6. Explain why fetal pulmonary vascular resistance is so high.

7. What percentage of blood entering the pulmonary artery actually flows through the lungs? Where does the rest of the blood go?

8. Describe the events that occur in the first few breaths after birth in terms of transpulmonary pressure, blood gases, and circulatory changes.

9. Compare the development of lung structures in newborns and adults.
   A. Number of alveoli

   B. Surface area of the lung

10. Compare the head and upper airway of adults and infants.

	ANATOMY	INFANTS	ADULT
A.	Head		
B.	Tongue		
C.	Nasal passages		
D.	Larynx		
E.	Narrow point		
F.	Dead space		
G.	Airways		

11. Most infants breathe exclusively through what part of the airway?

12. Explain why infant lung volumes are relatively lower than those of adults.

13. A. Grunting is a type of maneuver used by infants that is now known by what more modern term? B. What does it mean when an infant is grunting?

    A. _____

    B. _____

14. Why do infants experience severe hypoxemia more readily than adults?

Identify the structures labeled in these figures.

15. What's in a chest? Label the bones in this anterior view of the thorax.

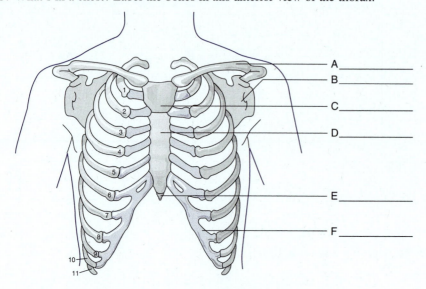

A_____

B_____

C_____

D_____

E_____

F_____

16. Label the imaginary lines on the anterior chest wall.

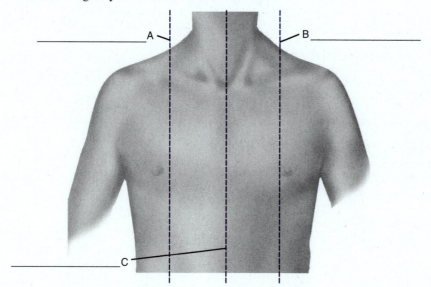

_____ A

B_____

_____ C

17. Label the imaginary lines on the lateral chest wall.

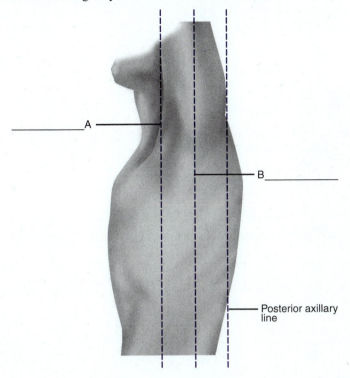

A _____

B _____

Posterior axillary
line

18. Identify and label the muscles of ventilation.

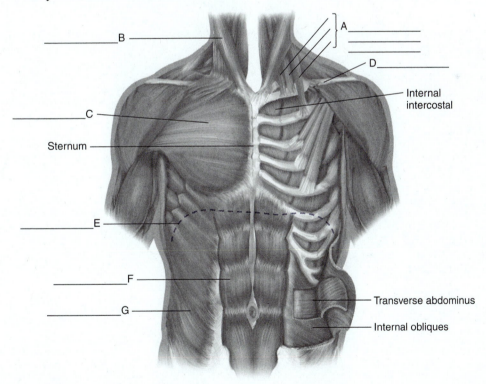

_____ B

_____ C

Sternum _____

_____ E

_____ F

_____ G

A _____
_____
_____

D _____

Internal
intercostal

Transverse abdominus

Internal obliques

19. Label the structures of the upper airway and oral cavity.

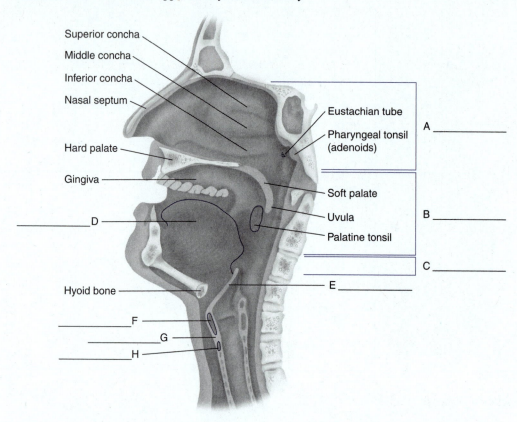

Superior concha

Middle concha

Inferior concha

Nasal septum

Eustachian tube

Pharyngeal tonsil (adenoids)

A _____

Hard palate

Gingiva

Soft palate

Uvula

B _____

Palatine tonsil

D _____

C _____

E _____

Hyoid bone

F _____

G _____

H _____

20. Label the anterior view of the larynx.

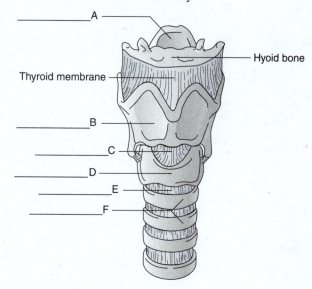

A _____

Hyoid bone

Thyroid membrane

B _____

C _____

D _____

E _____

F _____

21. Label the respiratory cilia.

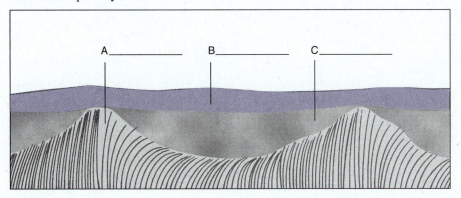

22. Label the cross-sectional sketch of the cells and organization of the alveolar septa.

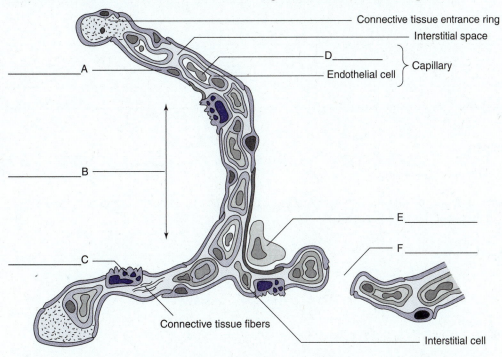

(From Hicks GH: Cardiopulmonary anatomy and physiology, Philadelphia, 2000, WB Saunders.)

LOBES AND SEGMENTS

Fill in the following chart.

	RIGHT LUNG		**LEFT LUNG**
	Right upper lobe		Left upper lobe
1.			Upper division
2.		1 and 2	
3.		3	
	Right middle lobe		Lower division (lingula)
4.		4	
5.		5	
	Right lower lobe		Left lower lobe
6.		6	
7.		7 and 8	
8.		9	
9.		10	
10.			

MEET THE OBJECTIVES

Fill in your answers in the spaces provided.

23. List the nerves that innervate the diaphragm, intercostal muscles, and larynx. State the origin of these nerves and describe what will happen if they are damaged.

24. Describe the pathway gas follows as it is conducted through the lower airway. Use Table 9-8 as a guide.

SUMMARY CHECKLIST

Fill in the spaces to identify eight key points from the Summary Checklist at the end of Chapter 9.

25. The _____ houses and protects the lungs.

26. The _____ is the primary muscle of ventilation.

27. The upper respiratory tract _____ and _____ inspired air and protects the lungs against _____ substances.

28. The lower respiratory tract _____ gases from the upper airway to the respiratory _____ of the lung.

29. The airways branch into _____, which are in turn made up of _____ in both the left and right lungs.

30. The respiratory bronchioles and _____ provide a large _____ for exchange of gases between air and blood.

CASE STUDIES

Case 1

A respiratory instructor tasks the students to learn the anatomy of the lung. Completely by coincidence, the instructor slips while running with scissors, and the sharp shears puncture his right chest. The students gather around their fallen facilitator to discuss the anatomic consequences of this tragedy.

31. What could happen to the lung on the affected side?

32. What could happen to the pleural space on the affected side?

33. What is this condition called?

34. What is the treatment for this condition?

Case 2

A registered respiratory therapist (RRT) is working the night shift at a large urban medical center. As he makes his rounds, he hears loud snoring coming from a patient's room. Even though snoring is a commonly heard sound at night, the RRT stops to investigate.

35. What anatomic change results in snoring?

36. What is OSA, and how is it treated?

37. What is the similarity between snorers and unconscious victims who require resuscitation?

38. How would you approach management of the airway of an unconscious person?

FOOD FOR THOUGHT

What happens to these structures when disease is present?

39. What happens to the airways and alveoli when a patient is having an acute episode of asthma?

40. What changes to the airways and alveoli occur in emphysema?

10 The Cardiovascular System

WORD WIZARD

Match the following terms to their definitions as they apply to respiratory care.

Terms	Definitions
_____ 1. Afterload	A. Membranous sac that surrounds the heart
_____ 2. Automaticity	B. Stroke volume multiplied by heart rate
_____ 3. Baroreceptors	C. Ventricular stretch provided by end-diastolic volume
_____ 4. Cardiac output	D. Biologic sensors that monitor arterial blood pressure
_____ 5. Chemoreceptors	E. Pathologic narrowing or constriction
_____ 6. Pericardium	F. Force against which the ventricle pumps
_____ 7. Preload	G. Biologic sensors that monitor arterial blood oxygen
_____ 8. Stenosis	H. Ability to initiate a spontaneous electrical impulse

MEET THE OBJECTIVES

9. Where is the mitral valve located? What effect can mitral valve stenosis have on the lungs?

10. Explain how specialized heart muscle tissue allows the muscle cells in the ventricle to contract in a coordinated and efficient manner.

11. Compare and contrast local control of blood vessels with central control mechanisms.

12. Describe how the cardiovascular system responds to exercise and blood loss by balancing blood volume and vascular resistance.

13. Match the mechanical events to their corresponding electrical events in the normal cardiac cycle.

	ELECTRICAL EVENT	CARDIAC EVENT (MECHANICAL)
A.	P wave	
B.	QRS	
C.	T wave	

SUMMARY CHECKLIST

Complete the following questions by writing the correct term(s) in the spaces provided.

14. The _____ system consists of the heart and vascular network, which maintain _____ by regulating the distribution of blood flow in the body.

15. Cardiac _____ is primarily determined by preload, _____, contractility, and

_____.

16. Under conditions of increased _____, special _____ mechanisms are called on to maintain stable flow.

17. The heart and vascular systems ensure that tissues receive sufficient blood to meet their _____ needs.

18. Blood pressure is regulated by changing the _____ of the blood, changing the _____ of the vascular system, or changing _____.

19. An increase in heart rate will likely cause a(n) _____ in cardiac output.

CASE STUDIES

Case 1

A 57-year-old patient is admitted to the coronary care unit with a diagnosis of mitral stenosis. The patient is breathing rapidly and complains of shortness of breath. Her pulse oximetry readings reveal hypoxemia. Auscultation reveals inspiratory crackles in the posterior lower lobes.

20. Describe mitral valve stenosis.

21. What mechanical events are occurring to cause pulmonary edema and stiffening of the lung tissue?

22. What action should the respiratory therapist take at this time?

Case 2

A respiratory care student is giving an aerosolized bronchodilator to a 27-year-old patient with asthma. Breath sounds reveal bilateral expiratory wheezing. The pulse oximeter shows 98% saturation on room air. The student notices the heart rate rising from 82 to 98 beats/min during the therapy.

23. What are the effects of sympathetic and parasympathetic stimulation on the sinus node in the heart?

    A. _____

    B. _____

24. Describe the two ways that drugs produce bronchodilation.

    A. _____

    B. _____

25. Based on this information, why would you expect increased heart rate to be a common side effect of drugs that cause bronchodilation?

WHAT DOES THE NBRC SAY?

Circle the best answer for the following questions.

26. A patient has a heart rate of 70 beats/min and a stroke volume of 60 ml with each contraction of the ventricle. What is the approximate cardiac output in liters per minute?
    A. 3.6 L/min
    B. 4.2 L/min
    C. 5.0 L/min
    D. 6.0 L/min

27. Calculate systemic vascular resistance if mean arterial pressure is 90 mm Hg, central venous pressure (CVP) is 10 mm Hg, and cardiac output is 4 L/min.
    A. 2.5 mm Hg/L/min
    B. 8.6 mm Hg/L/min
    C. 20 mm Hg/L/min
    D. 22.5 mm Hg/L/min

28. What is the ejection fraction if stroke volume is 50 ml and end-diastolic volume is 75 ml?
    A. 50%
    B. 66%
    C. 75%
    D. 150%

FOOD FOR THOUGHT

29. What four mechanisms combine to promote venous return to the heart?

    A. _____

    B. _____

    C. _____

    D. _____

30. What is meant by the "thoracic pump"? What effect can positive pressure ventilation, like CPAP, have on venous return to the chest?

11 Ventilation

WORD WIZARD

Complete the following paragraph by filling in the correct term(s) in the spaces provided.

Remember that the primary purpose of the lungs is to supply the body with oxygen and remove wastes in the form of carbon dioxide. _____ is the process of moving air in and out of the lungs. Some of that ventilation is _____ space, or wasted ventilation. When CO_2 builds up in the body, the pH of blood decreases, resulting in acidemia. We can measure the amount of air that moves in and out with a device called a spirometer. The pressure changes in the chest are measured using a body box, or _____. Finally, the actual rate of air flow is measured using a(n) _____. Airway _____ is a measurement of how much pressure it takes to push the gas through the conducting air passages. _____, or the distensibility (compliance), is the change in lung volume divided by the pressure needed to take that breath. Stiff lungs increase the work of breathing.

Much of respiratory care is aimed at reducing the work of breathing and restoring adequate ventilation. The process of respiration, on the other hand, is the exchange of gas between blood and other tissues.

PICTURE THIS

Label the following diagram to help improve your understanding of these pressure changes.

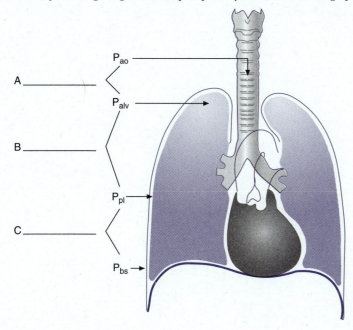

A _____

B _____

C _____

P_{ao}

P_{alv}

P_{pl}

P_{bs}

Pressures, volumes, and flows involved in ventilation. (Modified from Martin L: Pulmonary physiology in clinical practice: the essentials for patient care and evaluation, St. Louis, 1987, Mosby.)

1. Write out the definition of each gradient.

    A. Transrespiratory Pressure: _____

    B. Transpulmonary Pressure: _____

    C. Transthoracic Pressure: _____

Questions

2. Fill in the missing pressures for the apex and base of the lung.

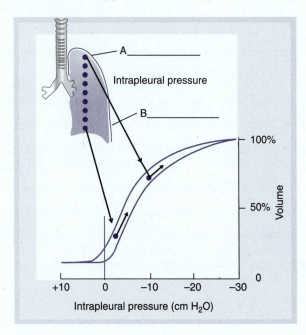

3. Where does the bulk of ventilation go during a normal breath in an upright person?

4. List the four factors that contribute to the work of breathing.

A. _____

B. _____

C. _____

D. _____

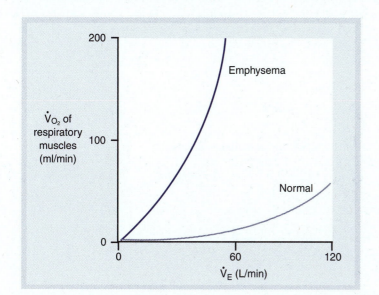

5. Why is the compliance of the lung tissue itself actually increased in emphysema?

6. What important change occurs in the airway of patients with COPD and asthma to increase the resistance? Which airways are usually involved?

7. What class of medications can respiratory therapists use to reduce airway resistance in asthma?

8. What does it mean when you see active exhalation in your patient?

9. What happens to persons with spinal cord injuries who cannot use their abdominal muscles?

10. Describe what happens to alveolar ventilation in healthy individuals when they increase respiratory rate or decrease tidal volume.

11. What is the optimal pattern of breathing for patients with obstructive airway diseases?

12. Label the types of dead space in this diagram.

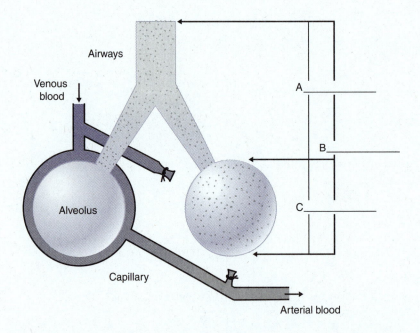

13. A. What is the normal percentage of anatomic dead space for each breath?
    B. What is the value used to calculate average anatomic dead space?

14. What type of ventilatory pattern will be seen with significantly increased dead space?

15. What is the difference between *hyperventilation* and *hyperpnea*?

16. Calculate exhaled minute ventilation for a patient who has a tidal volume of 800 ml and a frequency of 8 breaths/min.

    Formula _____

    Calculation _____

    Answer _____

17. Calculate anatomic dead space for a patient who is 6 feet tall and weighs 180 lb.

    Formula _____

    Calculation _____

    Answer _____

18. Calculate alveolar minute ventilation using the data from Problems 16 and 17.

    Formula _____

    Calculation _____

    Answer _____

19. Calculate the physiologic dead space using the Bohr equation if $PaCO_2$ is 60 mm Hg and $PECO_2$ is 30 mm Hg.

    Formula _____

    Calculation _____

    Answer _____

WHAT DOES THE NBRC SAY?

Circle the best answer for the following multiple choice questions.

20. The minute volume for a 68-kg (150-lb) patient who has a respiratory rate of 12 breaths/min and a tidal volume of 600 ml would be
    A. 4.8 L.
    B. 5.4 L.
    C. 6.0 L.
    D. 7.2 L.

21. The estimated alveolar minute ventilation for an 82-kg (180-lb) patient who has a respiratory rate of 10 breaths/min and a tidal volume of 500 ml would be
    A. 3.2 L.
    B. 3.5 L.
    C. 4.8 L.
    D. 5.0 L.

22. Which of the following ventilator settings would provide the optimal alveolar ventilation?

	Rate breaths/min	Volume ml
A.	10	600
B.	12	500
C.	15	400
D.	20	300

23. Determine the physiologic dead space percentage for a patient with an arterial CO_2 of 40 mm Hg and an exhaled CO_2 of 30 mm Hg.
    A. 0.25
    B. 0.33
    C. 0.50
    D. 0.75

12 Gas Exchange and Transport

4. If Patient B has an arterial PO_2 of 90 mm Hg, what is the A–a gradient?

Formula _____

Solution _____

Answer _____

5. Explain the difference in respiratory status between Patient A and Patient B based on the previous data.

6. List the three barriers to diffusion.

A. _____

B. _____

C. _____

7. What is the main force driving a gas across the alveolar-capillary membrane?

8. Calculate O_2 content for Patient 1 with an Hb of 15 g/dL, SaO_2 of 97%, and PaO_2 of 100 mm Hg.

Formula _____

Solution _____

Answer _____

9. Calculate O_2 content for Patient 2 with an Hb of 15 g, SaO_2 of 80%, and PaO_2 of 50 mm Hg.

Formula _____

Solution _____

Answer _____

10. Calculate O_2 content for Patient 3 with an Hb of 10 g, SaO_2 of 97%, and PaO_2 of 100 mm Hg.

Formula _____

Solution _____

Answer _____

Fill in the correct values for partial pressure of O_2 and saturation (with a normal pH) on the chart below. Use the Mini Clini on hemoglobin saturation (Page 256) if you need help.

	PaO$_2$	SaO$_2$
11.	40 mm Hg	
12.		80%
13.	60 mm Hg	
14.		97%

Fill in the correct answers for how the curve will shift in the following chart:

	Factor	Shift
15.	Acidosis	
16.	Hypothermia	
17.	High 2,3-diphosphoglycerate (2,3-DPG)	
18.	Fever	
19.	Hypercapnia	
20.	Carboxyhemoglobin	

GAS EXCHANGE

The following questions will test your knowledge of the causes of poor gas exchange.
Fill in the correct term(s) in the spaces provided.

21. Inadequate delivery of O_2 to the tissues is known as _____.

22. _____ is the medical name for a low level of O_2 in the blood.

23. Physiologic _____ occurs when blood passes through areas of the lung that have no ventilation.

24. Ventilation-_____ imbalances are the most common cause of low blood O_2 in patients with lung disease.

25. Patients with pulmonary fibrosis have a(n) _____ defect that results in low blood O_2 levels.

26. A low blood pressure results in _____ and poor tissue O_2 delivery.

27. Myocardial infarction is an example of _____, a localized reduction in blood flow to tissues that can result in tissue death.

28. Increased _____ space ventilation may result in increased levels of CO_2 in the blood.

29. Drug overdose may result in an inadequate _____ ventilation due to central nervous system depression.

30. Patients with severe COPD are unable to maintain adequate ventilation as a result of ventilation-_____ imbalances.

Circle the best answer for each of the following multiple choice questions.

31. A blood gas measurement in a patient breathing room air reveals the following results:

pH	7.50
$PaCO_2$	30 mm Hg
PaO_2	110 mm Hg

    In regard to these data, the respiratory therapist should
    A. report the results to the physician.
    B. redraw the sample because of air contamination.
    C. report that the patient is on O_2.
    D. place the patient on O_2.

32. Calculate O_2 content for a patient with the following data:

Hb	10 g
PaO_2	80 mm Hg
SaO_2	95%

    A. 12.73 ml O_2/dL
    B. 12.97 ml O_2/dL
    C. 13.40 ml O_2/dL
    D. 13.64 ml O_2/dL

33. Calculate PAO_2 for a patient with the following data:

P_B	747 mm Hg
FiO_2	0.21
PaO_2	95 mm Hg
$PaCO_2$	40 mm Hg
SaO_2	97%

    A. 97 mm Hg
    B. 103 mm Hg
    C. 107 mm Hg
    D. 117 mm Hg

34. A man is brought to the emergency department from a house fire. He is conscious and in obvious distress on 6 L of O_2 via nasal cannula. His heart rate is 135 beats/min, respiration is 26 breaths/min, and blood pressure is 160/100 mm Hg. The pulse oximeter reading is SpO_2 99% and heart rate is 136 beats/min. He has no cyanosis but complains of dyspnea. What abnormality of hemoglobin is most likely to be the source of the clinical problem?
    A. HbCO
    B. HbS
    C. Anemia
    D. HbF

CASE STUDIES

Case 1

A 29-year-old housewife is brought to the emergency department following exposure to smoke during a house fire. She is breathing at a rate of 30 breaths/min. Her heart rate is 110 beats/min. Blood pressure is 160/110 mm Hg. The patient complains of headache and nausea. The pulse oximeter reading shows a saturation of 99%.

35. Why are pulse oximeter readings unreliable in this setting?

36. What is wrong with this patient?

37. What action would you take at this time?

Case 2

A patient is brought back to the unit following major surgery after a motorcycle accident. He was given a massive blood transfusion to replace loss from both the trauma and the surgical procedure. The pulse oximeter reading is 96% on room air, but the nurse has requested your evaluation because of the patient's clinical condition. You find him sitting up and breathing 32 times per minute. He has tachycardia and tachypnea and complains of difficulty breathing. Breath sounds are clear on auscultation.

38. The patient's clinical signs are consistent with what gas exchange abnormality?

39. What is one of the potential problems with banked blood?

40. Name some of the other possible causes of the patient's distress.

41. What diagnostic procedure could you recommend?

Case 3

A woman is admitted with a diagnosis of pneumonia. Arterial blood gas measurements reveal a pH of 7.55, $PaCO_2$ of 25 mm Hg, PaO_2 of 75 mm Hg, and SaO_2 of 94%. She complains of feeling short of breath. Laboratory data reveal a hemoglobin level of 8 g/dL.

42. Interpret these blood gas findings in terms of gas exchange.

43. What other laboratory information plays a key role in helping to determine O_2 content?

44. What is absolute anemia, and how is it treated?

Case 4

A young man has been brought to the emergency department by paramedics after an accidental overdose of narcotics at a party. The patient is unconscious and has a respiratory rate of 8 breaths/min. The pulse oximeter shows a saturation of 85%.

45. Why would CO_2 be elevated in this patient?

46. Why is the patient's O_2 saturation so low?

SUMMARY CHECKLIST

47. The movement of gas between the lungs and the tissues depends mainly on _____.

48. The alveolar PCO_2 varies inversely with _____ ventilation.

49. _____ and _____ must be in balance to be effective.

50. Blood carries a small amount of dissolved O_2 in the plasma and a large amount carried in chemical combination with _____.

51. The five causes of a decreased PaO_2, or O_2, level in arterial blood are low ambient PO_2, _____, impaired _____, _____-_____ imbalances, and physiologic _____.

52. Most of the CO_2 in your blood is transported as _____.

53. Hypoxia can occur when _____ blood O_2 content is decreased or if blood _____ is decreased.

54. Alveolar ventilation decreases when the minute ventilation is _____ or when _____ ventilation is increased.

55. What is the classic example of dysoxia?

56. When does tissue O_2 consumption become dependent on O_2 delivery?

57. Why does lactic acid form when tissues are hypoxic?

13 Solutions, Body Fluids, and Electrolytes

WORD WIZARD

Write your answer in the spaces provided.

Definitions	Terms
1. _____ A compound that gives off H^+ in water.	A. Acid
2. _____ The opposite of inactive transport; movement across membranes.	B. Active transport
	C. Normal solution
3. _____ Negatively charged ion; Cl^- and HCO_3^- are common in the body.	D. Solvent
	E. Solute
4. _____ A compound that gives off OH^- in water.	F. Base
5. _____ Minimizing the change in pH.	G. Cations
	H. Hypertonic
6. _____ Positively charged ion; Na^+ and K^+ are common in the body.	I. Isotonic
7. _____ A substance with big molecules that hold water and also an evenly dispersed mixture or gel.	J. Solution
	K. Diluent
	L. Colloid
8. _____ Something you use to water down a medication or solution.	M. Dilute solution
9. _____ The medium you dissolve something into.	N. Hypotonic
10. _____ The stuff that gets dissolved.	O. Buffering
	P. Saturated solution
11. _____ A stable mixture of two substances. Heat helps make this happen.	Q. Anions
12. _____ A really weak solution.	
13. _____ A solution holding as much as it can.	
14. _____ The standard solution with 1 mEq/L.	
15. _____ Has the same amount of salt as your body fluids.	
16. _____ Saltier than your body fluids.	
17. _____ Low salt or no salt.	

WATER, WATER EVERYWHERE

18. Rank the relative amount of water in the following individuals. Put "1" by the group with the lowest percentage of body water and "5" by the group with the largest percentage of body water.

_____ Males

_____ Newborns

_____ Children

_____ Females

_____ Obese individuals

19. List subdivisions and give the relative amount (%) of water in each area.

COMPARTMENT	% H₂O
A. Intracellular	
B. Extracellular	
1.	
2.	
3.	

20. List the predominantly extracellular electrolytes.

A. _____

B. _____

C. _____

21. List the predominantly intracellular electrolytes.

A. _____

B. _____

C. _____

D. _____

22. What amount of water can be lost through fever?

23. Lost water is regained by two main methods. List these sources of liquids and give amounts.

	SOURCE	AMOUNT/DAY
A. Ingestion		
1.		
2.		
B. Metabolism		

ACID-BASE BASICS

24. If a patient ingested bicarbonate for stomach problems and the pH went up from 7.0 to 8.0, how much more alkaline did the body become?

25. What equation is used to calculate pH? Write it out to help remember it.

    A. Name

    B. Equation

ELECTRIFYING INFORMATION

26. List the seven major electrolytes and their primary purposes in the body.

	ELECTROLYTE	SYMBOL	PURPOSE
A.			
B.			
C.			
D.			
E.			
F.			
G.			

Match the value to the chemical in the list below.

27. _____ bicarbonate   A. 140 mEq/L

28. _____ calcium   B. 24 mEq/L

29. _____ chloride   C. 4.0 mEq/L

30. _____ magnesium   D. 5.0 mEq/L

31. _____ phosphorus   E. 100 mEq/L

32. _____ potassium   F. 2.0 mEq/L

33. _____ sodium   G. 1.4 mEq/L

Complete the chart below to match up disorders, causes, and symptoms of electrolyte disturbances.

	IMBALANCE	CAUSE	SYMPTOM
34.		Sweating	
35.	Hypokalemia		
36.		Starvation	Diaphragmatic weakness
37.	Hypercalcemia		
38.		Chronic renal disease	

CASE STUDIES

Case 1

A 68-year-old man with congestive heart failure (CHF) is being treated with a combination of diet and diuretics. He returns from a trip to New Orleans complaining of difficulty breathing and swollen ankles. He is admitted to the coronary care unit for observation and treatment. Auscultation reveals bilateral inspiratory crackles in the lung bases. His respiratory rate is 28 breaths/min, and his heart rate is 110 beats/min with arrhythmias. Hint: Check out the Mini Clini in the electrolyte section (Page 282).

39. Patients with CHF are usually placed on what special type of diet? Why?

40. Diuretics commonly cause loss of what specific electrolyte that affects cardiac function? How will this electrolyte be replaced in the hospital? The home?

    A. Electrolyte: _____

    B. Hospital replacement: _____

    C. Home replacement: _____

41. As a respiratory therapist, what action will you take to further assess cardiopulmonary status? What is likely to be your initial treatment of this patient?

42. What is the cause of this patient's lung crackles?

Case 2

A 68-year-old homeless alcoholic is found in respiratory distress by the paramedics and brought to your emergency department. The patient is malnourished. Auscultation reveals bilateral inspiratory crackles in the lung bases. His respiratory rate is 28 breaths/min with a heart rate of 110 beats/min. Hint: Look at the section on Starling equilibrium. We'll get back to these two cases again and again because pulmonary edema is such a common clinical problem; Chapter 29 is devoted to this topic. Now is a good time to get your feet wet in the area of flooded lungs.

43. What protein accounts for the high osmotic pressure of plasma? Why is this patient lacking this substance?

44. Explain why this patient has crackles.

45. As a respiratory therapist, what action will you take to further assess cardiopulmonary status? What is likely to be your initial treatment of this patient?

MATHEMATICS

46. Albuterol is prepared in a 5% solution (weight/volume). How many grams of albuterol are dissolved in 100 ml to make this solution?

    Formula _____

    Solution _____

    Answer _____

47. Respiratory therapists do not usually administer 100 ml of drugs to their patients. Instead, they give 1 ml or less. How many milligrams of albuterol would be found in 1 ml of the 5% solution in question 46?

    Formula _____

    Solution _____

    Answer _____

48. After drawing up 1 ml of a 5% solution of albuterol into a syringe, the respiratory therapist places the bronchodilator into a nebulizer along with 2 ml of saline for dilution. The total solution is now 3 ml in the nebulizer. What is the new concentration of the drug?

    Formula _____

    Solution _____

    Answer _____

Circle the best answer for each of the following multiple choice questions.

49. A patient with severe hypokalemia is receiving an intravenous infusion of potassium to correct this serious disorder. What should you monitor?
    A. SpO$_2$
    B. Respiratory frequency
    C. Mental status
    D. ECG rhythm

50. Which of the following signs and symptoms would you expect to observe in a patient with hypokalemia?
    1. Metabolic acid-base disturbance
    2. Muscle spasms and tetany
    3. ECG abnormality
        A. 1 only
        B. 1 and 2 only
        C. 1 and 3 only
        D. 2 and 3 only

51. All of the following would be consistent with administration of a large amount of IV fluid *except*
    A. increased pulmonary vascular markings on the chest x-ray.
    B. presence of crackles on auscultation.
    C. increased urine output.
    D. increased hematocrit.

52. A respiratory therapist delivers isotonic saline to a patient via nebulizer. What concentration of saline is the therapist delivering?
    A. 0.0%
    B. 0.45%
    C. 0.90%
    D. 1.0%

FOOD FOR THOUGHT

53. What happens to cells in the presence of a hypertonic solution?

54. What happens to cells in the presence of a hypotonic solution?

55. What is the name for the movement of water across a semipermeable membrane?

A medical student asked a respiratory therapist if the saline in his nebulizer treatment would hurt her patient, who was on sodium restriction for his heart. "No problem," said the RT. Use this scenario to answer the following question.

56. If you give 3 mL of normal saline by nebulizer, how much sodium chloride is being delivered to the airway in theory? Do you think the entire amount goes into the patient?

14 Acid-Base Balance

WORD WIZARD

Match the following terms to their definitions.

Terms	Definitions
1. _____ Acidemia	A. Acid that can be excreted in gaseous form
2. _____ Volatile acid	B. Decreased hydrogen ion concentration in the blood
3. _____ Anion gap	C. Ventilation that results in decreased CO_2
4. _____ Hyperventilation	D. Respiratory processes resulting in increased hydrogen ions
5. _____ Metabolic acidosis	E. Nonvolatile acid representing the byproduct of protein catabolism
6. _____ Alkalemia	F. Abnormal ventilator pattern in response to metabolic acidosis
7. _____ Kussmaul breathing	G. Nonrespiratory processes resulting in decreased hydrogen ions
8. _____ Hypoventilation	H. Difference between electrolyte concentrations
9. _____ Fixed acid	I. Respiratory processes resulting in decreased hydrogen ions
10. _____ Respiratory alkalosis	J. Increased hydrogen ion concentration in the blood
11. _____ Metabolic alkalosis	K. Nonrespiratory processes resulting in increased hydrogen ions
12. _____ Standard bicarbonate (HCO_3^-)	L. Chemical substance that minimizes fluctuations in pH
13. _____ Base excess	M. Plasma concentration of HCO_3^- corrected to a normal CO_2
14. _____ Respiratory acidosis	N. Difference between normal and actual buffers available
15. _____ Buffer	O. Ventilation that results in increased CO_2

WHERE HAS ALL THE ACID GONE?

16. Draw a diagram of the process called isohydric buffering.

Chapter **14 Acid-Base Balance**

17. Explain how the lungs can compensate for increased production of fixed acids.

18. Buffers are composed of what two components?

19. What happens when you add the acid hydrogen chloride to the base sodium bicarbonate?

20. What does ventilation remove from the body to help eliminate acid? Support your answer with information from the text.

21. Why are buffers in the kidney essential for the secretion of excess hydrogen ions?

BALANCING ACT

22. List the normal range of values for pH, $PaCO_2$, and HCO_3^-. (You MUST memorize these values!)

	Low Normal	High Normal
A. pH		
B. $PaCO_2$		
C. HCO_3^-		

23. Write out the Henderson-Hasselbalch equation.

24. Complete the primary acid-base and compensation chart below.

	Disorder	Primary Defect	Compensation
A.	Respiratory acidosis		
B.	Respiratory alkalosis		
C.	Metabolic acidosis		
D.	Metabolic alkalosis		

25. What is the "rule of thumb" for determining the expected increase in HCO_3^- for any acute increase in CO_2?

26. How much will HCO_3^- increase with a chronic increase in CO_2?

THE METHOD

There is a simple four-step method for interpreting blood gas values.

Step 1: Determine the pH first.
Step 2: Evaluate respiratory status ($PaCO_2$) to see if it agrees with the pH.
Step 3: Evaluate metabolic status (HCO_3^-) to see if it agrees.
Step 4: Evaluate compensation.

Interpret the following blood gas results.

27. pH   7.34
    $PaCO_2$ 60 mm Hg
    HCO_3^- 31 mEq/L

28. pH   7.36

     $PaCO_2$ 60 mm Hg

     HCO_3^- 33 mEq/L

Stop right there! We're going to continue interpreting blood gas results in the case studies and board examination review questions, but you can see how the HCO_3^- will be creeping up as the CO_2 rises and the pH returns to low normal to compensate.

THE ANION GAP

29. Name the three common causes of anion gap metabolic acidosis.

    A. _____

    B. _____

    C. _____

30. What are the signs of respiratory compensation for metabolic acidosis?

31. What are the neurologic symptoms of severe acidosis?

MATHEMATICS

32. Calculate the new HCO_3^- (assume 24 mEq/L as the starting point) level for an acutely elevated $PaCO_2$ of 70 mm Hg (assume it started at 40 mm Hg).

    Formula _____

    Solution _____

    Answer _____

33. Calculate the new HCO_3^- (assume 24 mEq/L as the starting point) level for a *chronically* elevated $PaCO_2$ of 70 mm Hg (assume it started at 40 mm Hg).

    Formula _____

    Solution _____

    Answer _____

34. Calculate pH if HCO_3^- is 30 mEq/L and $PaCO_2$ is 40 mm Hg.

    Formula _____

    Solution _____

    Answer _____

35. Calculate pH if HCO_3^- is 24 mEq/L and $PaCO_2$ is 40 mm Hg.

    Formula _____

    Solution _____

    Answer _____

36. Calculate pH if HCO_3^- is 24 mEq/L and $PaCO_2$ is 60 mm Hg.

Formula _____

Solution _____

Answer _____

37. Calculate anion gap if Na^+ is 144 mEq/ml, Cl^- is 100 mEq/ml, and HCO_3^- is 22 mEq/ml.

Formula _____

Solution _____

Answer _____

38. Calculate anion gap if Na^+ is 135 mEq/ml, Cl^- is 105 mEq/ml, and HCO_3^- is 26 mEq/ml.

Formula _____

Solution _____

Answer _____

CASE STUDIES

The following case studies will systematically take you through the major acid-base disorders. Let's start with some simple, acute states and move into the compensated ones. Remember to evaluate using the four-step process.

Case 1

Mrs. Betty Maladie was depressed and took too much diazepam (Valium). She is found *shortly* thereafter in a coma breathing slowly and shallowly. ABG results reveal pH of 7.28, $PaCO_2$ of 60 mm Hg, and HCO_3^- of 26 mEq/L.

39. How would you interpret this ABG?

40. What is the primary cause of the disorder?

Case 2

Mrs. M's husband, Bob, is very worried about her condition. He complains of dizziness and tingling in his hands. ABG results reveal pH of 7.58, $PaCO_2$ of 25 mm Hg, and HCO_3^- of 23 mEq/L.

41. How would you interpret this ABG?

42. What is the primary cause of the disorder?

The couple's young son, Billy, has been sick with the stomach flu. ABG results reveal pH of 7.60, $PaCO_2$ of 40 mm Hg, and HCO_3^- of 38 mEq/L.

43. How would you interpret this ABG?

44. What is the primary cause of the disorder?

Case 4

The couple's diabetic teenage daughter, Lizzy, has not been taking her insulin. ABG results reveal pH of 7.25, $PaCO_2$ of 40 mm Hg, and HCO_3^- of 17 mEq/L.

45. How would you interpret this ABG?

46. What is the primary cause of the disorder?

Of course, blood gases, like children, don't stay simple for long. Partial or complete compensation may occur.

Case 5

Grandpa Maladie has smoked for years, and now he has COPD. ABG results reveal pH of 7.37, $PaCO_2$ of 50 mm Hg, and HCO_3^- of 28 mEq/L.

47. How would you interpret this ABG?

48. What is the source of compensation?

Case 6

As soon as Lizzy Maladie's brain realizes the acute nature of her illness (Case 4), compensation begins. ABG results now reveal pH of 7.35, $PaCO_2$ of 25 mm Hg, and HCO_3^- of 13 mEq/L.

49. How would you interpret this ABG?

50. What is the source of compensation?

Grandma Maladie has congestive heart failure. She takes furosemide (Lasix) to reduce extra water in her body. ABG results now reveal pH of 7.46, $PaCO_2$ of 45 mm Hg, and HCO_3^- of 31 mEq/L.

51. How would you interpret this ABG?

52. What is a possible cause of the primary disorder?

WHAT DOES THE NBRC SAY?

Circle the best answer to the following multiple choice questions.

53. A 17-year-old girl is brought to the emergency department by paramedics. Her mother states she is a diabetic. Room air ABGs reveal the following:

pH	7.26
$PaCO_2$	16 mm Hg
HCO_3^-	8 mEq/L
PaO_2	110 mm Hg

This information indicates which of the following?
1. Partly compensated metabolic acidosis is present.
2. This PaO_2 is not possible on room air.
3. Respiratory alkalosis is present.
   A. 1 only
   B. 3 only
   C. 1 and 2 only
   D. 1 and 3 only

54. Interpret the following ABG results:

F_iO_2	0.21
pH	7.36
$PaCO_2$	37 mm Hg
HCO_3^-	22 mEq/L
PaO_2	95 mm Hg

A. Acute respiratory alkalosis
B. Acute metabolic alkalosis
C. Compensated respiratory alkalosis
D. Normal ABG

55. During CPR, blood gases are drawn. The results are as follows:

F_iO_2	1.0
pH	7.15
$PaCO_2$	55 mm Hg
HCO_3^-	12 mEq/L
PaO_2	210 mm Hg

What action should be taken to correct the acid-base abnormality shown here?
A. Increase the rate of ventilation.
B. Decrease the F_iO_2.
C. Administer sodium bicarbonate intravenously.
D. Add positive end-expiratory pressure (PEEP) to the ventilation system.

56. The results of an arterial blood gas measurement are as follows:

F_iO_2	0.21
pH	7.55
$PaCO_2$	25 mm Hg
HCO_3^-	24 mEq/L
PaO_2	105 mm Hg

These data indicate which of the following?
A. Metabolic acidosis
B. Metabolic alkalosis
C. Uncompensated hyperventilation
D. Uncompensated hypoventilation

57. A 72-year-old man with a history of renal failure is seen in the emergency department. The respiratory therapist notes that the patient is taking 28 very deep breaths per minute. Which of the following accurately describes this breathing pattern?
A. Cheyne-Stokes breathing
B. Ataxic breathing
C. Kussmaul breathing
D. Eupneic breathing

FOOD FOR THOUGHT

Blood gas disorders can get really complicated at times. In some cases, a patient will have one disorder superimposed on another.

Grandpa Maladie, discussed in Case 5, acquired a lung infection after visiting his daughter in the hospital. ABG results now reveal pH of 7.46 (pH previously 7.37), $PaCO_2$ of 55 mm Hg (previously 50 mm Hg), PaO_2 of 57 mm Hg, and HCO_3^- of 38 mEq/L (previously 28 mEq/L).

58. How would you interpret this ABG?

59. Why did the blood gas values change from those in the case?

15 Regulation of Breathing

WORD WIZARD

Finish the following sentences by filling in the correct terms.

1. _____ describes when there is no breathing at all.

2. Many important responses involve the vagus nerve and are called _____ reflexes.

3. The _____ center in the pons is ill defined, but gasping inhalations take place when it is out of control.

4. The _____ barrier prevents many substances from entering the cerebrospinal fluid.

5. The _____ center in the pons helps increase rate and control depth of ventilation and inspiratory time.

6. _____ respond to changes in O_2 and pH to signal the need to breathe.

CONTROL OF BREATHING

7. Label the parts of these central controlling bodies.

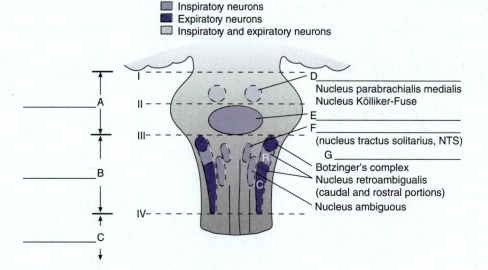

- Inspiratory neurons
- Expiratory neurons
- Inspiratory and expiratory neurons

D _____
Nucleus parabrachialis medialis
Nucleus Kölliker-Fuse
E _____
F _____
(nucleus tractus solitarius, NTS)
G _____
Botzinger's complex
Nucleus retroambigualis
(caudal and rostral portions)
Nucleus ambiguous

8. Briefly explain the role of the two primary respiratory groups in the medulla.

9. Compare and contrast the apneustic and pneumotaxic centers in the pons.

10. What diseases or conditions might affect the performance of the brainstem's respiratory controllers?

AUTOMATIC PILOT

Finish the following chart by filling in the correct terms.

	REFLEX	STIMULUS	RESPONSE	LOCATION
11.	Hering-Breuer			
12.	Deflation			
13.	Head			
14.	Vagovagal			
15.	C fiber			
16.	Proprioceptors			

CHEMICAL CONTROL OF BREATHING

17. Explain the process that allows CO_2 to stimulate the central receptors.

18. Describe the stimulating effects of CO_2 on the receptors in terms of the immediate response to increased CO_2 in the blood. What happens when this goes on for 1 or 2 days?

19. Describe the peripheral receptor response to decreased arterial O_2 levels. What do the receptors actually respond to when O_2 levels drop?

20. What specific range of PaO_2 values causes the greatest response when CO_2 and pH are normal?

21. How does altitude modify the receptor's response to hypoxemia?

22. Describe the peripheral receptor response to increased arterial CO_2 and H^+ ions. How is it different from the central chemoreceptor response?

23. What concentration of O_2 is usually given to chronically hypercapnic patients?

24. What is the best way to monitor oxygenation in these patients?

25. Why do low concentrations of O_2 usually result in adequate improvement?

26. Describe Cheyne-Stokes breathing (use words or draw a picture). State two important causes of this distinctive pattern.

27. How does Biot breathing differ from Cheyne-Stokes in terms of pattern and origin?

28. Describe apneustic breathing. What does this pattern indicate?

29. What are the two central neurogenic breathing patterns? State three events that could cause these patterns.

Case 1

Your patient rode his motorcycle without a helmet. He sustained a closed head injury during a crash that resulted in a subdural hematoma. The paramedics endotracheally intubated him and transported him to the emergency department.

30. Hyperventilation may lower the intracranial pressure of a patient with traumatic brain injury. What rules would you follow if you decide to do this procedure?
    A. When:
    B. Lowest safe CO_2 value:
    C. Length of time you can safely hyperventilate:

31. Why is lowering the CO_2 level controversial in traumatic brain injury?

Case 2

Grandpa Charlie, a COPD patient, is back in the hospital. He became short of breath at home, and his family increased his O_2 from 2 to 6 L/min. When he arrives at the hospital, he is somnolent and difficult to arouse. ABG results reveal that pH is 7.25, $PaCO_2$ is 75 mm Hg, PaO_2 is 90 mm Hg, and HCO_3^- level is 37 mEq/L on 6 L/min by nasal cannula.

32. What changes should you make in the patient's therapy? Why?

33. What target PaO_2 would be more appropriate for this patient? (Consider the PO_2 at which the receptors kick in.)

Circle the best answer for each of the following multiple choice questions.

34. A patient who has had COPD for many years is admitted for an acute episode of dyspnea. Arterial blood gas measured in the patient breathing room air gives these results:

pH	7.50
$PaCO_2$	48 mm Hg
PaO_2	44 mm Hg
HCO_3^-	36 mEq/L
SaO_2	84%

    What therapy do you recommend at this time?
    A. 28% Venturi mask
    B. 35% Venturi mask
    C. Nasal cannula delivering O_2 at 5 L/min
    D. Simple mask delivering O_2 at 10 L/min

35. A cooperative elderly patient with chronic asthma is examined at her pulmonologist's office. You observe the following findings:

Pulse	94 beats/min
RR	28 breaths/min
Temperature	36.5° C
BP	135/90 mm Hg
F_iO_2	0.21
pH	7.33
$PaCO_2$	70 mm Hg
PaO_2	35 mm Hg
HCO_3^-	34 mEq/L

    What action would you take at this time?
    A. Administer bronchodilator therapy via MDI and holding chamber.
    B. Administer O_2 via cannula at 2 L/min.
    C. Administer O_2 via cannula at 6 L/min.
    D. Administer O_2 via nonrebreathing mask.

36. A patient with COPD and a history of hypercapnia is receiving O_2 via simple mask at 10 L/min in the recovery room following admission for pneumonia. Upon transfer to the medical floor, he is noted to be increasingly drowsy and difficult to arouse. The nurse requests that you give him a breathing treatment with a bronchodilator. The most appropriate action would be to
    A. administer the breathing treatment as requested.
    B. obtain an arterial blood gas sample.
    C. change the O_2 to 2 L/min via nasal cannula.
    D. change the O_2 to 40% via Venturi mask.

37. A patient is being mechanically ventilated following craniotomy. During a suctioning procedure, the intracranial pressure monitor shows a sudden increase in intracranial pressure. The patient becomes restless and agitated. What is the most appropriate immediate action for the respiratory therapist in this situation?
    A. Increase the F_iO_2 on the ventilator to deliver 100% O_2.
    B. Recommend administration of a sedative.
    C. Increase rate and volume of ventilation with a resuscitation bag.
    D. Ask the registered nurse to page the physician "STAT."

EXPERIMENT

This exercise may seem simple, but it will help you understand control of breathing. It's even better if you have a pulse oximeter.

- Put the oximeter probe on your finger.
- Breathe normally.
- Now inhale deeply and hold your breath.
- Time how long you can hold your breath.
- Next, inhale and exhale deeply several times. Fill your lungs and time how long you can hold your breath. (Remember to be seated and have a partner.)
- Answer the following questions.

38. How long could you hold your breath the first time? _____ What about the second try?

_____

39. What were the pulse oximetry readings before _____, during _____, and at the end of breath holding?

40. Compare the results and explain the differences in the breath holding time and why you had to breathe. What is the meaning of the pulse oximetry readings?

SUMMARY CHECKLIST

41. Central chemoreceptors stimulate ventilation in response to the formation of _____ by CO_2 and water.

42. _____ increases the peripheral receptor response to arterial pH.

43. The primary stimulus for breathing in healthy individuals is arterial _____.

44. The secondary stimulus for breathing is arterial _____.

45. The breathing of patients with chronic hypercapnia is driven more by _____ stimulus than in patients with normal acid-base status.

46. _____ therapy is associated with acute arterial CO_2 retention in patients with

chronic _____.

FOOD FOR THOUGHT

47. Why do we measure patients' respiratory rates without telling them we are doing it?

48. Name as many factors as you can that involve the higher brain centers increasing the rate of ventilation.

49. An astronomy student goes to the volcano observatory (elevation 11,000 feet) for his first clinical assignment. What is likely to happen to his breathing pattern as he goes higher up the mountain? What causes this to happen?

50. What would happen over the next 24 hours and why?

16 Bedside Assessment of the Patient

WORD WIZARD

Match the following terms to their definitions as they apply to respiratory care.

Definitions	Terms
1. _____ Musical inspiratory or expiratory sound associated with asthma	A. Angina
2. _____ Difficulty breathing when lying supine	B. Barrel chest
3. _____ Shape of thorax associated with emphysema	C. Bradycardia
4. _____ Chest pain typical of acute coronary syndromes	D. Breathlessness
5. _____ Physical wasting associated with chronic lung disease	E. Cachexia
6. _____ Blood pressure that is too low	F. Crackles
7. _____ The sitting position that emphysema patients use when they are in trouble	G. Cyanosis
8. _____ Drop in blood pressure on inhalation associated with asthma and hyperinflation	H. Dyspnea
9. _____ Inspiratory sound associated with atelectasis, pneumonia, and fibrosis	I. Febrile
10. _____ Upper airway sound that may indicate life-threatening obstruction	J. Orthopnea
11. _____ Soft tissue sucking in around ribs and neck when a patient has severe distress	K. Pulse deficit
12. _____ Dizziness associated with drop in blood pressure	L. Pulse pressure
13. _____ A rapid heart rate that may indicate a low blood oxygen level	M. Pulsus paradoxus
14. _____ Presence of a fever	N. Retractions
15. _____ Difference between systolic and diastolic blood pressure	O. Shock
16. _____ A slow heart rate that may result in poor perfusion of tissues	P. Stridor
17. _____ Bluish discoloration of skin often associated with hypoxemia	Q. Syncope
18. _____ Heart rate auscultated in chest is different than pulse rate felt in arm	R. Tachycardia
19. _____ Difficulty breathing	S. Tripoding
20. _____ Sensation of suffocation	T. Wheezes

21. What information would you gather before entering the patient's room?

22. Describe how to *start* the ideal interview. Be sure to discuss space, privacy, and introductions.

    A. Space: _____

    B. Privacy: _____

    C. Introductions: _____

23. Circle the *best approach* from each set of choices in the following list:
    A1. "Hi, Bob, good morning."
    A2. "Good morning, Mr. Johnson."

    B1. Stand at the foot of the bed.
    B2. Sit in a chair at the bedside.

    C1. Make room for your notes on the bedside table.
    C2. Keep your clipboard on your lap.

    D1. "Do you need anything right now?"
    D2. "I'll tell your nurse to check on you."

    E1. "I'll be back to see you in one hour."
    E2. "I'll return in a while to check on you."

24. Circle the best approach from each set of choices in following list:
    A1. "What are you coughing up?"
    A2. "You didn't cough up blood, did you?"

    B1. "I understand you don't like your breathing treatments."
    B2. "Why don't you like these treatments?"

    C1. "How is your breathing today?"
    C2. "Is your breathing better today?"

25. When are "closed" questions most useful? Give an example.

26. Describe the dyspnea (Borg) scale. List several reasons why this scale would be useful.

27. How else can you identify the degree of dyspnea a patient feels? Explain the difference between dyspnea and breathlessness.

28. What are the possible causes of these common types of cough?

	Cough	Cause(s)
A.	Dry	
B.	Loose, productive	
C.	Acute, self-limiting	
D.	Chronic	

29. What is the difference between mucus and sputum?

30. What are the three characteristics of sputum that should be documented and reported to the physician and other members of the health care team?

31. What is the most serious kind of nonpleuritic chest pain?

32. How does pleuritic chest pain differ from nonpleuritic pain?

33. Significant elevation of temperature will have what result on metabolic rate, oxygen consumption, carbon dioxide production, and breathing pattern?

34. Along with fever, what are two signs that are highly suggestive of respiratory infection?

A. _____

B. _____

MEDICAL HISTORY

35. What do the initials "CC" and "HPI" stand for? List at least five important areas described in the HPI.

A. CC = _____

B. HPI = _____

    1. _____

    2. _____

    3. _____

    4. _____

    5. _____

36. What do the initials "PMH" stand for? List at least five important areas described in the PMH.

A. PMH = _____

    1. _____

    2. _____

    3. _____

    4. _____

    5. _____

37. Describe the significance of the findings for each of the areas of general appearance listed below.

	FINDING	SIGNIFICANCE
1.	Weak, emaciated, and diaphoretic	
2.	Appears anxious	
3.	Sitting up, leaning with arms on table	

38. What does the phrase "oriented × 3" mean?

39. Compare and contrast the terms "lethargic" and "obtunded."

40. What is the difference between a "stuporous" patient and a "comatose" patient?

41. What is the first thing a respiratory therapist should evaluate in cases of a depressed level of consciousness?

VITAL INFORMATION

42. Fill in the correct normal values (or terms) for an adult in the chart below.

	SIGN	AVERAGE NORMAL	LOWEST NORMAL	HIGHEST NORMAL
A.	Temperature			
B.	Heart rate			
C.	Respiratory rate			
D.	Systolic blood pressure			
E.	Diastolic blood pressure			

43. Match these terms to their definitions.

Terms	Definitions
A. Bruits	1. Palpable vibrations in pulse
B. Amplitude	2. Strength of pulse
C. Paradoxical pulse	3. Drop in amplitude with inspiration
D. Pulsus alternans	4. Alternating strong and weak pulses

44. Match these respiratory patterns to their definitions.

Patterns	Definitions
A. Tachypnea	1. Difficulty breathing in a supine position
B. Eupnea	2. Abnormally low respiratory rate
	3. Deep breathing
C. Platypnea	4. Normal breathing pattern
D. Hyperpnea	5. Abnormally high respiratory rate
	6. Labored breathing in an upright position
E. Bradypnea	

45. How can you prevent patients from becoming aware (and consciously altering) that you are taking their respiratory rate?

46. What does it mean when patients show a larger (> 6 to 8 mm Hg) than normal drop in systolic pressure during inspiration?

47. Write a description for the following six abnormal chest shapes.

Abnormal chest shape	Description
A. Barrel	_____
B. Kyphosis	_____
C. Kyphoscoliosis	_____
D. Pectus carinatum	_____
E. Pectus excavatum	_____
F. Scoliosis	_____

48. Explain the difference between vocal and tactile fremitus.

49. Describe the difference between fremitus in emphysema and in pneumonia.

50. How does subcutaneous emphysema form? What is the feeling of air under the skin called?

51. Complete the following chart by identifying the percussion notes for the conditions.

Condition	Percussion Note
A. Emphysema	_____
B. Atelectasis	_____
C. Pleural effusion	_____
D. Pneumothorax	_____
E. Pneumonia	_____

52. What are the limitations of percussion? What can't you palpate?

53. Fill in the chart below with descriptions of your favorite breath sounds.

	BREATH SOUND	PITCH	INTENSITY	LOCATION
A.	Vesicular			
B.	Bronchial			
C.	Bronchovesicular			

54. Compare the mechanisms and causes of coarse, low-pitched crackles and fine, end-inspiratory crackles.

55. Contrast monophonic and polyphonic wheezes in terms of mechanisms, phase of ventilation, and conditions that produce these different musical sounds.

56. How do you test for capillary refill? What is a normal capillary refill time?

57. Where should you check for edema caused by heart failure? Why?

58. Answer the following questions about cyanosis.

A. What is the specific cause of cyanosis? _____

_____

B. What is peripheral cyanosis? _____

_____

C. What is the main cause of peripheral cyanosis? _____

_____

CASE STUDIES

Case 1

An alert 67-year-old politician is admitted for dyspnea and hemoptysis. While interviewing the patient you discover that he has been coughing up small amounts of thick, blood-streaked mucus several times per day for the last few days. He has a history of 100 pack-years of cigarette smoking. Physical examination reveals a barrel chest, use of accessory muscles, and digital clubbing.

59. The patient's history and chest configuration suggest what primary pulmonary disorder?

60. Along with enlargement of the ends of the fingers, what sign helps you recognize clubbing?

61. What does the presence of clubbing suggest in this case?

A 47-year-old female is admitted for a systemic infection 3 days after cutting herself in the kitchen while preparing some chicken. She complains of dyspnea and has a fever. Her vital signs are pulse 110 beats/min, respiratory rate 28 breaths/min, and blood pressure 76/58 mm Hg. The nurse's notes reveal that the patient was alert on admission, but she is now confused and anxious. Her extremities are warm and capillary refill is normal.

62. Why do you think the patient's mental status has deteriorated?

63. What other "vital sign" should be evaluated?

64. Which abnormal vital sign has the most clinical significance in this case?

A 59-year-old rock star is recovering from open heart surgery performed 2 days earlier. He is alert and oriented × 3. He complains of dyspnea and a dry cough. Vital signs reveal a pulse of 104 beats/min and a respiratory rate of 32 breaths/min with a shallow pattern. The patient tells you that his difficulty breathing started yesterday and has been gradually getting worse. Auscultation reveals decreased breath sounds in both bases with end-inspiratory crackles.

65. What is the most likely cause of the dyspnea?

66. What diagnostic test is indicated to confirm the diagnosis?

67. What respiratory care intervention(s) is indicated?

WHAT DOES THE NBRC SAY?

68. There are vibrations on exhalation over the upper chest. What action should be taken at this time?
    A. The patient should be given a bronchodilator.
    B. The patient should be suctioned.
    C. The patient should be given supplemental oxygen.
    D. The patient should be placed on mechanical ventilation.

69. A patient's medical record indicates that he has orthopnea. Which of the following best describes this condition?
    A. Difficulty breathing at night
    B. Difficulty breathing when upright
    C. Difficulty breathing on exertion
    D. Difficulty breathing when lying down

70. A child is brought to the emergency department for severe respiratory distress. Upon entering the room, the RT hears a high-pitched sound when the child inhales. This is most likely
    A. wheezing.
    B. stridor.
    C. rhonchi.
    D. crackles.

71. An RT is asked to evaluate a patient for oxygen therapy. She notices that the patient is sleepy but arouses when questioned. This level of consciousness is best described as
    A. confused.
    B. obtunded.
    C. stuporous.
    D. lethargic.

72. During an interview, the patient states he has been coughing up thick, foul-smelling sputum. This finding is most consistent with
    A. a bacterial infection of the lung.
    B. a diagnosis of lung cancer.
    C. obstructive lung disease.
    D. pulmonary tuberculosis.

73. An RT is inspecting the chest of a child with respiratory distress. The practitioner notes that the child has a large concave depression of the sternum. This finding should be documented as
    A. barrel chest.
    B. pectus carinatum.
    C. pectus excavatum.
    D. kyphoscoliosis.

17 Interpreting Clinical and Laboratory Data

WORD WIZARD

Because the following words sound so similar, it's easy to get confused. *Leuko* means "white," *erythro* means "red," and *thrombo* means "blood clot"—at least they do in Latin. Now use these in filling in some of the spaces below.

_____ is the study of blood. The CBC, or complete _____ _____, is a test used to establish the overall picture of the blood. A _____ test value is significantly outside the normal range and may be life threatening to the patient. White blood cells are called _____. When the white blood count goes up in infection, we call it _____. If the white count goes down, it is called _____. Hemoglobin is found in the _____ and can carry oxygen. Your blood won't clot without the smallest formed element, the _____. A condition of _____ may result in bleeding if you suction or draw a blood gas!

LAB TESTS

1. What does a large elevation in white blood cell (WBC) count suggest?

   A. _____

   B. _____

   C. _____

2. List three common causes of low WBC count.

   A. _____

   B. _____

   C. _____

3. What specific type of WBC is elevated in bacterial pneumonia? Viral pneumonia?

   A. Bacterial: _____

   B. Viral: _____

4. Which WBCs are involved in problems such as allergic asthma?

5. What term describes a low red blood cell (RBC) count? What is the treatment for this disorder?

    A. Term: _____

    B. Treatment: _____

    _____

6. What is a normal hemoglobin level, and why are RTs especially interested in hemoglobin levels?

    A. Normal: _____

    B. Respiratory role: _____

    _____

7. What blood abnormality is caused by chronic hypoxemia?

8. Before performing an arterial blood gas (ABG), you would be wise to check which two *specific* laboratory values?

    A. Blood count _____

    B. Blood chemistry test _____

9. What is the normal range for serum potassium?

10. Why is potassium of particular interest in patients being weaned from mechanical ventilation?

11. Give at least one clinical example of how a patient develops a very high or very low potassium level.

    A. Hyperkalemia _____

    B. Hypokalemia _____

12. What value on the venous chemistry panel represents bicarbonate?

13. Low chloride levels occur for what two primary reasons?

    A. _____

    B. _____

14. Why is the chloride level in sweat so important? What is the critical value?

    A. Importance: _____

    B. Value: _____

15. What other test is indicated when a chemistry panel shows an abnormal anion gap?

16. What are the two tests that together indicate renal function?

17. Name the two common liver enzymes that might be elevated in patients with hepatitis.

    A. _____

    B. _____

18. CPK is an example of an enzyme that can show you specific injury to brain, lungs, heart, or muscles. Describe the three types of CPK and what they mean.

    A. CPK-BB _____

    B. CPK-MM _____

    C. CPK-MB _____

19. Discuss troponin I and explain why it would be important in emergency medicine.

20. Another interesting chemical can tell you if the patient has heart failure, rather than a heart attack. What does BNP stand for and how do we use this test?

    A. BNP = _____

    B. What does it show us? _____

    C. Name another condition that can elevate BNP. _____

21. What is PT?

    A. Full name _____

    B. When is it used? _____

22. What is PTT?

    A. Full name _____

    B. When is it used? _____

    C. Explain the difference in the two tests.

    D. Name medications associated with PTT.

23. Explain the D-dimer test and how it is useful to respiratory therapists.

24. What blood cell is vital to clotting, and what is its normal value?

25. Why would the laboratory reject your beautiful sputum specimen? Give specific reasons and include numerical values.

   A. Pus _____

   B. Epithelial cells _____

   How can you improve the quality? Have patients rinse out their mouth and pharynx before you have them cough.

26. What is the purpose of growing the bacteria on a culture plate?

CASE STUDIES
Case 1

A patient presents in the emergency department complaining of shortness of breath, fever, and productive cough. A chest radiograph reveals pneumonia in the right lower lobe.

27. What blood test is indicated?

28. What specific finding would suggest bacterial pneumonia?

29. What would you like to do about the sputum?

A 60-year-old, two-pack-per-day smoker has a complete blood count ordered, and his WBC count is 9000. His hematocrit is 60%, and his hemoglobin is 20 g/dL.

30. What is the name for this elevation of red blood cells?

31. What respiratory problem is indicated by the high hematocrit and hemoglobin?

WHAT DOES THE NBRC SAY?

32. Sputum culture and sensitivity would be indicated for which of the following conditions?
    A. ST segment elevation
    B. Pleural effusion
    C. Pneumothorax
    D. Bronchitis

33. A patient presents in the emergency department with vomiting. Blood gas results reveal metabolic alkalosis. Based on this information, you would also suggest
    A. a STAT chest radiograph.
    B. an electrolyte analysis.
    C. a complete blood count.
    D. clotting time.

34. A Chem 7 panel was ordered for a patient in the emergency department and hypokalemia is present. What test should the RT recommend?
    A. STAT chest radiograph
    B. Arterial blood gas
    C. Sputum culture
    D. Complete blood count

35. A sputum culture that is sent to the lab is likely to be rejected as saliva if
    A. fewer than 25 epithelial cells are present.
    B. fewer than 25 pus cells are present.
    C. more than 25 epithelial cells are present.
    D. more than 25 pus cells are present.

FOOD FOR THOUGHT

36. A young adult male patient presents with symptoms of hypoxemia and signs of pneumonia. What are several possible reasons the WBC count is severely depressed?

ANATOMY OF THE IMPULSE-CONDUCTING SYSTEM OF THE HEART

Label all the heart parts and conduction clues.

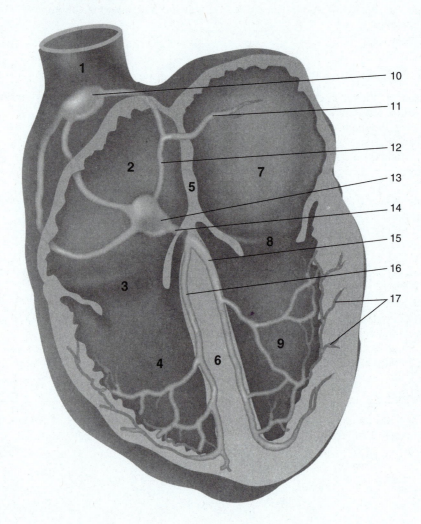

Heart Parts	Conduction Clues

Heart Parts

1. _____

2. _____

3. _____

4. _____

5. _____

6. _____

7. _____

8. _____

9. _____

Conduction Clues

10. _____ Natural "pacemaker" of the heart

11. _____ Conducts impulses through the atria

12. _____ Carries impulses across the right atrium

13. _____ "Backup pacemaker"

14. _____ Bundle of cardiac fibers that conducts impulses that regulate the heartbeat

15. _____ Carries impulse to the left ventricle

16. _____ Carries impulse to the right ventricle

17. _____ Finger-like projections that penetrate the ventricles

18. Identify the normal configuration of electrocardiograph waves, segments, and intervals along with what they represent in the spaces below.

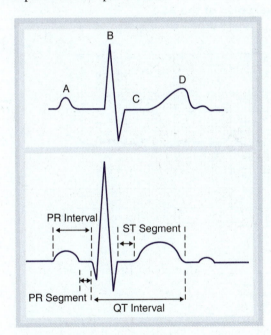

Wave, segment, and intervals

A. P wave

B. QRS complex

C. ST segment

D. T wave

Represents

_____

_____

_____

_____

Now answer the following questions about ECG waves.

19. Where is atrial repolarization?

20. What is the maximum duration of the P–R interval?

21. What pathologic abnormality results in a depressed or elevated ST segment?

MAKING MEASUREMENTS

22. What is the normal paper speed for an ECG?

23. The time (horizontal axis) represented by one small box is _____ seconds and by one large box is _____ seconds.

24. One millivolt of electrical energy will produce a deflection of _____ small boxes or _____ large boxes.

Successful ECG interpretation begins with a systematic evaluation of the ECG.
Step 1: Evaluate the Rate

25. The number of QRS complexes in this 6-second strip is _____ Multiply by 10 to get a rate of _____.

26. There are _____ heavy lines between complex A and complex B; 300 divided by this number is _____. That's the average rate!

    Is every P wave followed by a QRS complex? That indicates a sinus rhythm!

27. If the rate is below 60 beats/min, it is called sinus _____.

28. If the rate is above 100 beats/min, it is called sinus _____.

Step 2: Measure the P–R Interval

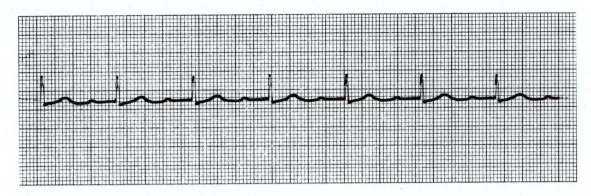

29. The time from the P wave to the QRS complex is _____ second(s).

30. What arrhythmia does this represent?

Step 3: Evaluate the QRS Complex

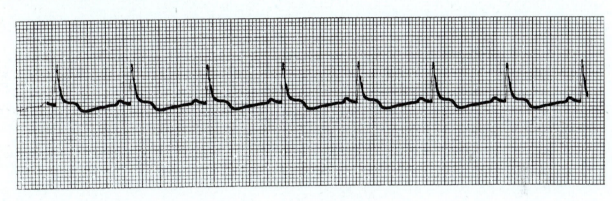

31. The duration of the QRS complex is _____ second(s).

Step 4: Evaluate the T Wave

32. The T wave in pattern 1 is (circle one)

    upright

    inverted

Step 5: Evaluate the ST Segment

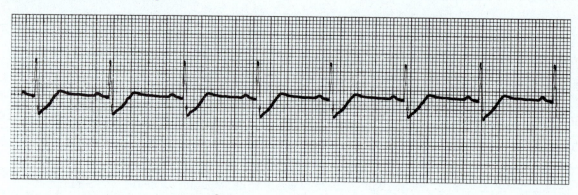

33. The ST segment in pattern 4 is (circle one)
    elevated
    flat
    depressed

Step 6: Identify the RR Interval

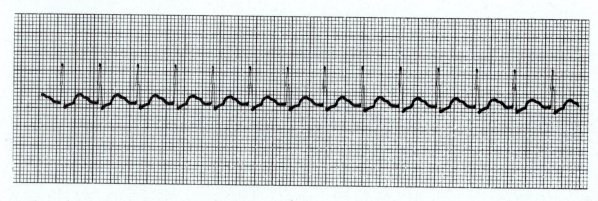

34. The RR interval in this pattern is (circle one)
    regular
    irregular

CASE STUDIES

Case 1

A student is suctioning a patient orally with a tonsil suction. The monitor shows sinus bradycardia. Blood pressure is falling. Alarms are sounding.

35. What should the student do?

36. What physiologic mechanism was responsible for the drop in rate?

A student is suctioning a patient via the endotracheal tube. The monitor shows sinus tachycardia with frequent premature ventricular contractions. Alarms are sounding. The patient is agitated.

37. What should this student do about the arrhythmias?

38. What physiologic mechanism was responsible for the increased rate and arrhythmias?

While performing a ventilator check on a patient in the coronary care unit, a student observes the rhythm on the monitor has changed from atrial fibrillation to ventricular fibrillation.

39. What should the student do first?

40. Name at least three responses indicated to treat this rhythm.

WHAT DOES THE NBRC SAY?

Circle the best answer.

41. An RT is suctioning a patient on a ventilator and observes the following rhythm on the monitor:

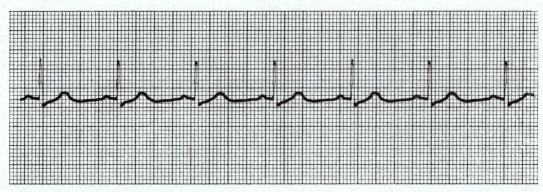

In regard to this pattern, the RT should
A. continue to suction the patient.
B. stop and administer 100% oxygen.
C. recommend atropine administration.
D. defibrillate the patient.

42. An RT is preparing to perform an arterial puncture when the following rhythm is observed on the monitor:

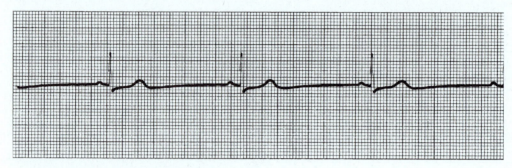

In regard to this pattern, the RT should
A. continue to suction the patient.
B. stop and administer 100% oxygen.
C. recommend atropine administration.
D. defibrillate the patient.

43. During a routine suctioning procedure, an RT notes the following rhythm on the cardiac monitor:

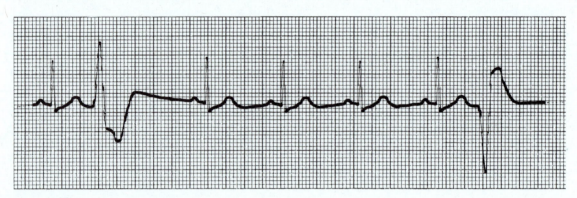

In regard to this pattern, the RT should
A. continue to suction the patient.
B. stop and administer 100% oxygen.
C. recommend atropine administration.
D. defibrillate the patient.

44. During a routine suctioning procedure, an RT notes the following rhythm on the cardiac monitor:

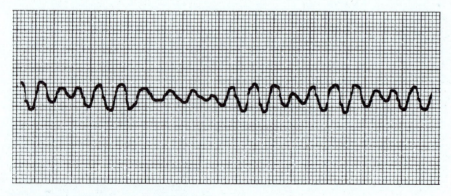

In regard to this pattern, the RT should
A. continue to suction the patient.
B. stop and administer 100% oxygen.
C. recommend atropine administration.
D. defibrillate the patient.

45. A respiratory therapist is called to perform a STAT ECG on a patient with chest pain in the emergency department. Proper placement of chest lead V6 is the
   A. fourth intercostal space, left sternal margin.
   B. fourth intercostal space, right sternal margin.
   C. fifth intercostal space, left midaxillary line.
   D. fifth intercostal space, left midclavicular line.

FOOD FOR THOUGHT

46. Have you ever had to disrobe at the physician's office or clinic? How did you feel? How do you think patients feel when you ask them to disrobe?

47. How will you ensure that your patients don't feel awkward or embarrassed when you do ECGs or chest exams?

19 Analysis and Monitoring of Gas Exchange

WORD WIZARD

Match the following quality terms to their definitions.

Definitions	Terms
1. Examining the repeatability of results.	A. Quality control
2. Comparing the values with a known value.	B. Bias
3. Errors of precision.	C. Imprecision
4. Another term associated with errors of precision.	D. Random error
5. A trend or abrupt shift in data outside the limits.	E. Systematic error
6. An oblique or diagonal line.	F. Preanalytical error
7. Problems that occur prior to testing a sample.	G. Precision
8. CLIA standards are an important example.	H. Accuracy

MEET THE OBJECTIVES

Answer the following questions.

9. In your own words, explain how an electrochemical analyzer converts the number of O_2 molecules (PO_2) into a measurable reading.

10. Name the two common types of electrochemical analyzers.

    A. _____

    B. _____

11. Explain the differences between the two types of analyzers in terms of principle of operation and response time.

12. Describe the two-step process for calibrating an O_2 analyzer.

13. What is the gold standard of gas exchange analysis? What does this mean?

14. List four reasons that explain why the radial artery is the preferred site for ABG sampling.

    A. _____

    B. _____

    C. _____

    D. _____

15. Describe the modified Allen test and give the definition of a positive result.

    A. _____

    B. _____

16. Name four other sites you can use if the radial artery is unavailable or has a poor pulse.

    A. _____

    B. _____

    C. _____

    D. _____

17. How long should you wait after changing the F_iO_2 before performing an ABG on a patient with healthy lungs? A patient with COPD?

    A. _____

    B. _____

18. Name the four things you can do to avoid most preanalytical sampling errors.

    A. _____

    B. _____

    C. _____

    D. _____

19. What precaution should you take when handling any laboratory specimen?

20. If you wanted to measure actual hemoglobin saturation, what type of analyzer would be needed?

21. What is the range of accuracy for most commercially available pulse oximeters?

22. Describe three noninvasive ways you can determine the reliability of a pulse oximeter at the bedside.

    A. _____

    B. _____

    C. _____

23. According to the AARC guidelines, what action should you take to verify the results when pulse oximetry is unreliable or does not confirm suspicions about the patient's clinical state?

24. What are the two most common errors committed during capillary sampling?

    A. _____

    B. _____

25. Explain what variables are reliable and unreliable in capillary sampling compared to arterial sampling.

26. What are the primary advantages and disadvantages of transcutaneous gas monitoring over arterial sampling?
    A. Advantages

        1. _____

        2. _____

    B. Disadvantages

        1. _____

        2. _____

27. When would you choose a pulse oximeter for monitoring an infant's oxygenation status over a transcutaneous monitor?

28. When would the transcutaneous monitor be preferred over the pulse oximeter?

29. What are the normal values for end-tidal CO_2 for healthy individuals and how do they compare with values for arterial CO_2?

30. An end-tidal CO_2 of "0" may indicate a serious problem. Name two life-threatening causes of a "0" value for end-tidal CO_2.

    A. _____

    B. _____

31. While performing end-tidal CO_2 measurements, you notice that the baseline does not return to "0" on inspiration. Interpret this result.

32. While performing end-tidal CO_2 measurements, you notice that no real plateau is reached. Give two possible interpretations of this result.

    A. _____

    B. _____

SUMMARY CHECKLIST

33. What are the three most common causes of O_2 analyzer malfunctions?

    A. _____

    B. _____

    C. _____

34. Blood gases provide more information than other methods of gas exchange analysis. What are the three general areas that a blood gas helps to assess?

A. _____

B. _____

C. _____

35. What is the maximum ideal time between ABG sampling and analysis?

36. What are the two primary benefits and hazards of indwelling peripheral arterial lines?
A. Benefits

1. _____

2. _____

B. Hazards

1. _____

2. _____

37. What is point-of-care testing, and what are the potential benefits of this method of testing blood samples? Name a potential problem or drawback.

38. What is the difference between capnography and capnometry?

39. Indwelling arterial, central venous, or pulmonary artery catheters are widely used in the ICU. Please list the two main benefits and two main drawbacks of these invasive lines.
A. Benefits

B. Drawbacks

Case 1

A 34-year-old firefighter is brought to the emergency department for treatment of smoke inhalation while fighting a house fire. His heart rate is 126 beats/min, and respirations are 28 breaths/min and labored. SpO_2 is 100% on 6 L/min via nasal cannula. Blood pressure is 145/90 mm Hg. Breath sounds are coarse with inspiratory crackles in both bases. The patient's face is smudged with soot, and he is coughing up sputum with black specks in it.

40. What clinical signs of hypoxemia does the patient display?

41. Explain why the pulse oximeter is reading 100% despite these signs.

42. What is the most probable cause of the hypoxemia?

43. What blood test would you recommend to confirm your suspicions?

Case 2

A premature infant is receiving supplemental O_2. Her physician is concerned about the effects of hyperoxia on her lungs and eyes. The infant is being monitored by a pulse oximeter, which shows a saturation of 100%.

44. What range of PaO_2 is possible with an SpO_2 of 100%?

45. What type of noninvasive monitoring would you recommend in this situation?

Case 3

An elderly patient is admitted for acute exacerbation of his long-standing COPD. He is wearing a nasal cannula with a flow rate of 2 L/min.

46. What is the simplest way to quickly assess his oxygenation status?

47. Why would you recommend arterial blood gas sampling for this patient?

Case 4

A patient was riding his motorcycle without a helmet when he crashed. Now he has a head injury and is being mechanically ventilated. His physician asks you to make recommendations regarding monitoring his gas exchange.

48. What are the advantages of using capnometry to monitor carbon dioxide in this situation?

49. Where would you place the capnometer probe in the ventilator circuit?

50. During monitoring, you notice that the capnograph does not return to "0" when the patient inhales. What does this indicate?

51. A few minutes later, the patient's exhaled CO_2 levels begin to rise. So does his blood pressure. The patient becomes agitated. What action would you take?

52. Why do rising CO_2 levels cause increases in intracranial pressure?

WHAT DOES THE NBRC SAY?

Circle the best answer.

53. A respiratory therapist is preparing to perform pulse oximetry. Which of the following would be *least* beneficial for assessing accuracy of the device?
    A. Checking the capillary refill time
    B. Assessing skin color and temperature
    C. Performing an Allen test on the patient
    D. Assessing pulse rate

54. Which of the following would you perform after obtaining an arterial blood gas sample?
    1. Remove air bubbles from the sample.
    2. Mix the sample by rotating the syringe.
    3. Maintain site pressure for at least 1 minute.
    4. Add heparin to the sample.
        A. 1 only
        B. 1 and 2 only
        C. 1, 2, and 3 only
        D. 1, 2, 3, and 4

55. A pulse oximeter is being used to monitor a patient who was rescued from a fire. The SpO_2 is 90%; however, the patient is unconscious and shows signs of respiratory distress. What additional test should the RT recommend?
    A. CT scan
    B. Electrolyte measurement
    C. Co-oximetry
    D. Hemoglobin and hematocrit levels

Chapter **19** Analysis and Monitoring of Gas Exchange

56. A polarographic O_2 analyzer fails to calibrate when exposed to 100% O_2. The first action the respiratory therapist should take would be to
    A. replace the battery.
    B. replace the membrane.
    C. replace the fuel cell.
    D. try another O_2 source.

57. An infant is placed on a transcutaneous O_2 monitor. The $TcPO_2$ is reading 40 mm Hg less than the PaO_2 obtained from an arterial sample. All of the following could cause this problem *except*
    A. improper calibration of the transcutaneous electrode.
    B. room air contamination of the transcutaneous electrode.
    C. inadequate heating of the skin at the electrode site.
    D. inadequate perfusion of the skin at the electrode site.

58. Which of the following analyzers is calibrated to a value of zero when exposed to room air?
    A. Clark electrode
    B. Galvanic O_2 analyzer
    C. Capnometer
    D. Geisler type of nitrogen analyzer

59. Which of the following would be most useful in assessing proper tube placement following endotracheal intubation?
    A. Transcutaneous monitoring
    B. Arterial blood gas analysis
    C. Pulse oximetry
    D. End-tidal CO_2 monitoring

60. Complications of arterial puncture include all of the following *except*
    A. pulmonary embolus.
    B. hematoma.
    C. infection.
    D. nerve damage.

61. A galvanic O_2 analyzer is being used as a check of the ventilator system to measure the delivered F_iO_2. The set F_iO_2 is 40%; however, the analyzer is reading 32%. Which of the following is the most likely cause of this discrepancy?
    A. The batteries in the analyzer need to be changed.
    B. The electrode membrane has water condensation on its surface.
    C. The analyzer needs to be calibrated.
    D. The ventilator requires servicing.

62. Which of the following will affect the accuracy of pulse oximeter measurements?
    1. Increased bilirubin levels
    2. Decreased hematocrit levels
    3. Dark skin pigmentation
    4. Exposure to sunlight
        A. 1 and 2 only
        B. 2 and 3 only
        C. 3 and 4 only
        D. 2, 3, and 4 only

63. An arterial blood gas sample is drawn from a patient who is breathing room air. Analysis reveals the following results:

pH	7.45
$PaCO_2$	35 mm Hg
PaO_2	155 mm Hg

    Which of the following best explains these results?
    A. Too much heparin was added to the sample.
    B. An air bubble has contaminated the sample.
    C. Analysis of the sample was delayed for more than 60 minutes.
    D. The patient was hyperventilating during the puncture.

64. Which of the following sites would be the best for continuous monitoring of exhaled carbon dioxide during mechanical ventilation?
   A. Exhalation valve
   B. Inspiratory side of the ventilator circuit
   C. Expiratory side of the ventilator circuit
   D. Endotracheal tube connector

65. Which of the following is true concerning the use of a transcutaneous PO_2 monitor?
   A. $TcPO_2$ should be checked with arterial blood samples.
   B. The skin temperature control should be maintained at 37° C.
   C. The site should be changed every 24 hours.
   D. The low calibration point is determined using room air.

FOOD FOR THOUGHT

66. How would you modify your technique if you had to perform ABGs on a patient receiving anticoagulants?

67. Why can you use a capnometer during CPR but not a pulse oximeter?

20 Pulmonary Function Testing

Match the right terms or abbreviations with the correct definition.

Terms/Abbreviations	Definitions
1. DLCO	A. Volume inspired with a normal breath.
2. ERV	B. Greatest amount of air you can breathe in 12 to 15 seconds.
3. VT	C. Largest amount of air the lungs can hold.
4. IRV	D. Fastest flow rate generated at the very beginning of forced exhalation.
5. RV	E. Milliliters of gas the lung can transfer to the blood.
6. TLC	F. Amount of air you can exhale after a maximum inspiration.
7. VC	G. Ratio of volume exhaled in 1 second to total volume exhaled.
8. IC	H. Average expiratory flow during the early part of forced exhalation.
9. FRC	I. Amount of air you can inhale after a normal exhalation.
10. MVV	J. Amount of air you can inhale after a normal inspiration.
11. FVC	K. Air left in the lungs after a maximum exhalation.
12. PEF	L. Air left in the lungs after a normal exhalation.
13. $FEF_{200-1200}$	M. Amount of air you can forcefully exhale after a maximum inspiration
14. FEV_1	N. Average expiratory flow during the middle part of forced exhalation.
15. $FEF_{25\%-75\%}$	O. Volume of air you can forcefully exhale in 1 second.
16. FEV_1/FVC	P. Amount of air you can exhale after a normal exhalation.

Put the four lung volumes and four lung capacities into perspective with their normal values in a healthy adult. Use the box provided. MEMORIZE this information! It will serve you well on your board examinations!

A	E	C	B
	F		
	G	D	
	H		H

17. Fill in the names and normal values that go with each letter in the box.

	VOLUME/CAPACITY	VALUE
A.		
B.		
C.		
D.		
E.		
F.		
G.		
H.		

MEET THE OBJECTIVES

Answer these questions to find out if you have grasped the important points for each area of lung testing.

Lung Volumes

18. Which volumes *cannot* be measured with a spirometer?

19. Which capacities *cannot* be measured with a spirometer?

20. Name the three tests used to determine the volumes and capacities that cannot be measured.

A. _____

B. _____

C. _____

21. What is thoracic gas volume?

22. How will volumes or capacities obtained by helium dilution or nitrogen washout differ from those obtained with a body plethysmograph for a patient with air trapping?

23. What effect will an air leak have on the values obtained by helium dilution or nitrogen washout?

Spirometry

24. What four variables are used to calculate normal values for spirometry?

A. _____

B. _____

C. _____

D. _____

25. You must produce acceptable results that provide valid, reliable information based on how long the patient exhales, how closely multiple tests correlate, and how fast the patient starts the maneuver. Fill in the details for each of the criteria below:

A. Duration: _____

B. Variance of two best FVCs: _____

C. Satisfactory start: _____

D. Minimum number: _____

26. Which FVC should you report? Which FEV_1?

    A. FVC: _____

    B. FEV_1: _____

27. Which flow rate is the greatest?

28. Which flow rate represents large airways?

29. Which flow rate represents the middle range?

30. A spirometer is considered accurate if the volume is verified to be within what percentage of a known value?

31. What device is used to verify the volume of a spirometer?

32. What is the normal value for MVV? How is this test performed?

Diffusion

33. What gas is usually used to measure the lung's ability to transfer gas to the blood?

34. What other special gas is used in this test? Why?

35. What blood test results are needed to ensure accuracy of diffusion studies?

INTERPRETATION FUNDAMENTALS

36. There are two major categories of pulmonary disease. Fill in the chart below to compare the effects of each category.

	CATEGORY	ANATOMY	PHASE	PATHOLOGIC CONDITION	MEASURE
A.	Obstructive				
B.	Restrictive				

37. Fill in the corresponding percentage of predicted values for the degrees of impairment.

Degree of Impairment	% Predicted Value
Normal	_____
Mild	_____
Moderate	_____
Severe	_____

38. The original normal values for pulmonary functions were probably based on a 6-foot-tall, 20-year-old white male. How are normal values corrected for nonwhites?

39. Compare the FEV_1/FVC ratios you would see in normal, obstructed, and restricted patients.

A. Normal: _____

B. Obstructed: _____

C. Restricted: _____

CASE STUDIES

Case 1

Spirometry is performed on a 24-year-old woman who complains of a "tight chest" and cough. Simple spirometry shows the following:

Test	Actual	Predicted	% Predicted
FVC	3.2 L	4 L	80%
FEV_1	1.6 L	3.2 L	50%
FEV_1/FVC	50%	70%	

40. Interpretation?

41. What test should be performed in light of the results and the clinical information? (If you're not sure, check out PFT Report No. 2 in the Mini Clini that starts on page 425.)

Case 2

A 34-year-old respiratory care student is required by his instructor to undergo pulmonary function testing as part of a course. Here are the results:

Test	Actual	Predicted	% Predicted
FVC	3.9 L	4.8 L	81%
FEV_1	3.1 L	4.1 L	76%
FEV_1/FVC	79%	70%	

42. Interpretation?

43. What pulmonary function test would you suggest performing now?

Case 3

A 60-year-old shipyard worker complains of dyspnea on exertion and dry cough. Here are his spirometry results.

Test	Actual	Predicted	% Predicted
FVC	2 L	4 L	50%
FEV_1	1.5 L	3.4 L	44%
FEV_1/FVC	75%	70%	
TLC	2.4	4.8	50%

44. Interpretation?

45. What additional test would be helpful?

46. What additional history would be helpful?

Case 4

A woman in her physician's office complains of dyspnea on exertion. Spirometry and lung volume results show the following.

Test	Actual	Predicted	% Predicted
FVC	1.5 L	3 L	50%
FEV_1	0.75 L	2.5 L	30%
FEV_1/FVC	50%	70%	
TLC	2.6 L	3.8 L	68%

47. Interpretation?

48. What additional history would be helpful?

A 70-year-old man with a 100-pack-year smoking history complains of a dry cough and dyspnea on exertion. Results of lung tests show the following.

Test	Actual	Predicted	% Predicted
FVC	2.9 L	4.4 L	65%
FEV_1	1.3 L	3.7 L	35%
FEV_1/FVC	59%	70%	
TLC	6.6 L	5.5	120%
FRC	4.5 L	2.2	
RV	3.7 L	1.1 L	
DLCO	16	25	64%

49. Interpretation? Be complete; what specific type of disease is suggested?

50. What disease state do the lung volumes and history suggest?

51. Why is the vital capacity lower than predicted?

For additional practice, be sure to check out the case studies in Chapter 19 of your textbook!

WHAT DOES THE NBRC SAY?

Circle the best answer.

52. Which of the following tests would be helpful in assessing the effects of cigarette smoking on the smaller airways?
    A. FVC
    B. $FEF_{25\%-75\%}$
    C. FEV_1
    D. $FEF_{200-1200}$

53. A patient's physician asks you to recommend a pulmonary function test to help assess the effects of a possible tumor in the trachea. Which of the following would you recommend?
    A. Spirometry with volume-time curves
    B. Spirometry before and after bronchodilator
    C. Lung volume studies via nitrogen washout
    D. Spirometry with flow-volume loops

54. A pulmonary function technologist tests a spirometer by injecting 3.0 L of air from a large-volume syringe. The spirometer measures 2.90 L. Which of the following is true regarding this situation?
    A. The results are within normal limits.
    B. The spirometer is not ready to use.
    C. The air was injected too slowly.
    D. The BTPS corrections were not made properly.

55. Which of the following values could be incorrectly calculated?

Test	Actual	Predicted	% Predicted
FVC	4.4 L	4.8 L	92%
FEV_1	3.5 L	4.1 L	80%
FEV_1/FVC	80%	70%	
TLC	5.2 L	5.5	
FRC	2 L	2.4	
ERV	1.2 L	1.2 L	
RV	1 L	1.2 L	

    A. TLC
    B. FVC
    C. FRC
    D. RV

56. Which of the following pulmonary measurements is usually the smallest?
    A. Inspiratory capacity
    B. Vital capacity
    C. Functional residual capacity
    D. Total lung capacity

57. The following results were obtained from spirometry of an adult female smoker with chronic bronchitis. What is the correct interpretation?

Test	Actual	Predicted	% Predicted
FVC	3.9 L	4.8 L	81%
FEV_1	3.1 L	4.1 L	76%
FEV_1/FVC	79%	70%	

    A. Results indicate a mild diffusion defect.
    B. Results are within the normal range.
    C. A mixed obstructive/restrictive defect is present.
    D. Results show obstructive lung disease.

---

*In *Egan's* you will find the answer under the topic of reversibility. Unfortunately, the new ATS standard is 12% and at least 200 ml. The boards will give a hearty increase in reversible cases so you don't get confused.

Chapter **20** **Pulmonary Function Testing**

58. After a bronchodilator is administered, what percentage increase in forced spirometric volumes or flow rates is the *minimum* indication that reversible airway obstruction is present?[*]
   A. 5%
   B. 10%
   C. 15%
   D. 20%

59. Which of the following can be measured during spirometric testing?
   A. Residual volume
   B. Tidal volume
   C. Total lung capacity
   D. Functional residual capacity

60. An increased total lung capacity combined with a decreased diffusing capacity is strongly indicative of which of the following conditions?
   A. Emphysema
   B. Pneumonia
   C. Pulmonary fibrosis
   D. Pleural effusion

FOOD FOR THOUGHT

We have just scratched the surface of a complex area of testing. Entire textbooks are devoted to pulmonary function testing! Here are a few more questions to fill up the corners of your brain.

61. What effect does smoking have on the results of a diffusion test? Why?

62. What lung volume or capacity is useful in predicting normal values for incentive spirometry?

21 Review of Thoracic Imaging

WORD WIZARD

Complete the following paragraphs by writing the correct term(s) in the spaces provided.

The chest _____, or as it is more commonly called, the chest film or x-ray, is one of the most common methods for evaluating the lungs and other structures in the thorax. Air-filled lung tissue appears mostly dark on the film

because it is easily penetrated by x-rays. We describe this effect by saying the tissue is _____. The dense bone

tissue of ribs appears white. Dense matter that is not easily penetrated is referred to as _____. Fat is dense so it appears whiter than air or tissues. A female patient's breast tissue will alter the appearance of film. Obesity has the same effect. Soft tissues such as blood vessels appear more grayish because they have an intermediate density.

Abnormal conditions may be spotted through observation of certain densities in the wrong location. Accumulation of

fluid in the pleural space, or _____, appears white and may obscure the angle where the ribs meet the dia-

phragm. If pus collects in the pleura, we call it _____. Alveoli appear white when filled with pus or blood.

On the chest film these white areas are called pulmonary _____. If alveoli are filled with fluid but the airways

around them are open, you will see air _____ that may indicate pneumonia. Air in the pleural space, or a

_____, is another example of an abnormal density. This condition appears as a black area with none of the usual grayish markings of blood vessels in the lung tissue.

OVERVIEW

1. Describe the four tissue densities you can see on a chest radiograph.

   A. Air: _____

   _____

   B. Fat: _____

   _____

   C. Tissue: _____

   _____

   D. Bone: _____

   _____

2. Physicians may order, but RTs recommend; we all work toward good care of the patient. Name three indications for a chest radiograph.

Outpatient (clinic or office setting)

A. _____

B. _____

C. _____

Inpatient (ED, ICU, or medical/surgical patient)

A. _____

B. _____

C. _____

3. Explain "lag" in reference to the chest x-ray.

STEP-BY-STEP

4. The two basic ways to shoot a plain chest film are anterior to posterior (AP) and posterior to anterior (PA). You'll want to know which method was used before you continue your evaluation. Explain the differences between AP and PA.
   A. Where does the film go in relationship to the chest, and where is the energy beam (x-ray machine)?
      1. PA

      2. AP

   B. What might happen to the heart in an AP film?

   C. If PA films are so much better in quality, why do most of our patients have AP chest x-rays?

5. What structures offer clues to help identify whether the patient's position is straight or rotated?

6. What appearance of the vertebral bodies suggests underexposure?

7. What effect does underexposure have on the appearance of lung tissue?

8. The pleura appear at the edge of the chest wall (although the pleura themselves are usually difficult to see). What are the two major pleural abnormalities detected on the chest film?

A. _____

B. _____

ADVANCED CHEST IMAGING

9. CT = _____

What's the advantage over regular radiographs?

What is CT angiography used for?

10. HRCT = _____

Explain the concept of "slices" and what this technique is good for showing.

11. MRI = _____

What type of tissue in the chest is imaged with this technique?

IDENTIFYING ABNORMALITIES

Evaluation of the Pleura

12. What is the costophrenic angle?

13. Describe how you recognize the presence of fluid in the pleural space; what does that angle look like?

14. Which view is most sensitive for detecting pleural fluid? How is the patient positioned to obtain this view?

15. When is sonography (ultrasound) indicated in the evaluation of pleural abnormalities?

16. What other imaging procedure may be helpful?

17. Air in the pleural space is always abnormal. Name three common causes of this condition.

    A. _____

    B. _____

    C. _____

18. What breathing maneuver will help identify a small pneumothorax on a chest film?

19. Tension pneumothorax is immediately life threatening. Name at least two radiographic signs of tension pneumothorax.

    A. _____

    B. _____

20. What is the treatment for tension pneumothorax?

Evaluation of Lung Parenchyma

21. What are the two components of the lung parenchyma?

    A. _____

    B. _____

22. How will alveolar infiltrates appear on the chest film?

23. What is the difference between the radiographic appearance of pneumonia and pulmonary hemorrhage?

24. What causes airways to become visible, and what is this sign called?

25. Honeycombing, nodules, and volume loss are all radiographic hallmarks of what type of lung disorder?

26. Describe the silhouette sign. Discuss the difference between a right lower lobe and right middle lobe infiltrate as seen on a chest film.

Pathologies

27. List some of the causes of pulmonary edema.

    Vascular

    A. _____

    B. _____

    C. _____

28. Describe Kerley B lines. When do you see them?

29. What are "bat's wings"?

Lost Volume

30. List five important indirect signs of volume loss, or atelectasis, seen on the chest radiograph.

    A. _____

    B. _____

    C. _____

    D. _____

    E. _____

31. You can count on the ribs to tell you about lung volumes. Fill in the chart below based on which anterior ribs you would see above the diaphragm depending on the degree of lung inflation.

	LUNG VOLUME	ANTERIOR RIBS
A.	Poor inspiration	
B.	Good effort	
C.	Hyperinflation	

32. Ribs aren't the only way to assess COPD with hyperinflation. List the two primary and three secondary radiographic signs seen in emphysema.

A. Primary

1. _____

2. _____

B. Secondary

3. _____

4. _____

5. _____

33. Compare the sensitivity of the chest radiograph and computed tomography for detection of obstructive airway disease.

Catheters, Lines, and Tubes

Checking placement of tubes and lines is key for RTs.

34. The endotracheal tube is made of soft plastic. How can the chest film be useful in deciding correct tube position after intubation?

35. In an ideally placed endotracheal tube, where is the distal tip in relation to the carina?

36. Where will the endotracheal tube usually end up if it is placed too far into the trachea?

37. What pulmonary complication may be identified on a chest film when a CVP catheter is placed via the subclavian vein?

38. A pulmonary artery catheter (Swan-Ganz) that is seen to extend too far into the lung fields of a chest radiograph may have what unwanted results?

135

The Mediastinum

39. Where does the mediastinum lie within the chest?

40. What imaging technique is most favored for assessing mediastinal masses?

CASE STUDIES

Case 1

You are asked to perform postural drainage and clapping on a patient with a large right-sided pulmonary infiltrate. Evaluation of the chest radiograph shows a patchy white density with air bronchograms in the right lung. The right border of the heart is visible in the film.

41. Based on your knowledge of the silhouette sign, in what lobe is the infiltrate located?

42. What diagnosis does the presence of air bronchograms suggest?

43. What physical assessments could confirm the information in the chest film?

Case 2

An elderly man presents in the emergency department with acute exacerbation of his long-standing COPD. A decision is made to intubate him. It is difficult to auscultate breath sounds, and chest movement is minimal; however, your impression is that breath sounds are more diminished on the left. A chest radiograph is obtained, which shows the tip of the endotracheal tube 1 cm above the carina. The left lung field is slightly smaller than the right. Both diaphragms appear flat, and you are able to count eight anterior ribs above the diaphragms.

44. Where should the tip of the tube be in relation to the carina?

45. With regard to the endotracheal tube, what action should you take?

46. What is the significance of the flattened diaphragms and number of ribs seen above the diaphragm?

Circle the best answer.

47. A patient has dyspnea and tachycardia following thoracentesis to treat a pleural effusion. Evaluation of this patient

    should include a(n) _____ .
    A. CT scan
    B. MRI
    C. chest radiograph
    D. bronchoscopy

48. A pneumothorax would appear on a chest radiograph as a _____.
    A. white area near the lung base
    B. white area that obscures the costophrenic angle
    C. dark area without lung markings
    D. dark area with honeycomb markings

49. The medical record of an intubated patient indicates that the morning chest film shows opacification of the lower right lung field with elevated right diaphragm and a shift of the trachea to the right. These findings suggest

    _____.
    A. left-sided pneumothorax
    B. right-sided pleural effusion
    C. right mainstem intubation
    D. right-sided atelectasis

50. On a chest radiograph, the tip of the endotracheal tube for an adult patient should be _____.
    A. 2 cm above the vocal cords
    B. 2 cm above the carina
    C. at the carina
    D. 2 cm below the carina

51. A patient is believed to have a pleural effusion. Which of the following radiographic techniques would be most useful in making a confirmation?
    A. CT
    B. Decubitus radiograph projection
    C. MRI
    D. AP radiograph projection

52. What specific type of chest radiograph may be useful in evaluating pleural effusion?
    A. Lateral decubitus position
    B. Apical lordotic position
    C. Lateral upright
    D. PA expiratory film

53. A patient with a history of hypertension presents in the ED with headache, slurred speech, and left-sided weakness. What diagnostic imaging procedure would the respiratory therapist recommend to further evaluate this patient according to the ACLS guidelines?
    A. Computed tomography (CT)
    B. Ultrasound
    C. Angiography with contrast
    D. Magnetic resonance imaging (MRI)

54. A patient with a history of pulmonary pathology and cancer presents with a suspicious mediastinal mass on the chest x-ray. What diagnostic imaging procedure would be useful in gathering further information about the mass?
    A. Computed tomography (CT)
    B. Ultrasound
    C. Angiography with contrast
    D. Magnetic resonance imaging (MRI)

55. Ultrasound is useful in the cardiopulmonary setting for
    1. guiding catheter placement.
    2. evaluation of pleural effusion.
    3. evaluation of pneumonia.
    4. diagnosis of myocardial infarction.
        A. 1 and 2 only
        B. 1 and 3 only
        C. 2 and 4 only
        D. 3 and 4 only

56. A respiratory care practitioner is treating a child with respiratory distress in the emergency department. Which type of diagnostic imaging procedure may be useful for differentiating between epiglottitis and croup in children?
    A. AP chest x-ray
    B. Lateral neck x-ray
    C. MRI
    D. Ultrasound

57. The respiratory therapist is checking a patient-ventilator system in the medical intensive care unit when the high-pressure alarm begins to sound. Breath sounds are absent on the left with good tube placement. Blood pressure is 80/50 mm Hg. SpO_2 is 86% and falling. The heart rate is 160 beats/min. There is a hyperresonant percussion note on the left upper chest. The patient has lost consciousness. What action should the respiratory therapist take at this time?
    A. Call for a STAT portable chest x-ray.
    B. Remove the patient from the ventilator and begin manual ventilation.
    C. Remove the endotracheal tube and begin manual ventilation.
    D. Recommend immediate needle decompression of the chest.

FOOD FOR THOUGHT

58. The author states that patient head position is important in assessing the placement of the tip of an endotracheal tube on a radiograph. What happens to the tube if the head moves up (extension) or the chin goes down (flexion)? How far can the tube move?

22 Flexible Bronchoscopy and the Respiratory Therapist

FLEXIBLE BRONCHOSCOPY

1. List five clinical situations where flexible bronchoscopy (FB) would be indicated.

    A. _____

    B. _____

    C. _____

    D. _____

    E. _____

2. List three absolute and relative contraindications for FB.
    Absolute contraindications

    A. _____

    B. _____

    C. _____

    Relative contraindications

    A. _____

    B. _____

    C. _____

3. What is the goal of sedation during FB?

4. Describe the Mallampati classification.

5. List three vital sign measurements the respiratory therapist should monitor while a patient is sedated for an FB. What else should be monitored?

A. _____

B. _____

C. _____

DIAGNOSTIC BRONCHOSCOPY

6. What is a BAL and when is it indicated?

A. BAL: _____

B. Indication: _____

7. What is the difference between a BAL and bronchial washings?

THERAPEUTIC BRONCHOSCOPY

8. When is rigid bronchoscopy (RB) indicated?

THERMAL ABLATION OF THE ENDOBRONCHIAL LESION

9. Describe the following thermal ablation techniques.

A. Electrocautery: _____

B. Argon plasma coagulation: _____

C. Laser photocoagulation: _____

10. What are the above techniques used for?

11. What should a respiratory therapist consider regarding oxygen delivery during thermal ablation?

12. What are endobronchial stents used for?

13. Describe the two different types of endobronchial stents.

 A. _____

 B. _____

14. List two indications for a self-expanding metallic stent.

 A. _____

 B. _____

EMERGING BRONCHOSCOPIC INTERVENTIONS

15. What patient population may benefit from bronchial thermoplasty (BT)?

CASE STUDY

You are the respiratory therapist (RT) in the intensive care unit (ICU) of a large urban trauma center. You are about to assist the physician with an FB procedure on an intubated patient who is receiving mechanical ventilation.

16. What preprocedure responsibilities are the RT accountable for to ensure patient safety?

17. What vital signs would you be evaluating during the procedure? Is there anything else the respiratory therapist may assist with during the procedure?

18. What serious complications are possible following this type of procedure?

WHAT DOES THE NBRC SAY?

Circle the best answer.

19. You are preparing a patient for her flexible bronchoscopy procedure. Her weight is 50 kg. What is the total dose of lidocaine that should not be exceeded to help avoid methemoglobinemia?
    A. 300 mg
    B. 350 mg
    C. 400 mg
    D. 450 mg

20. What effects could be seen during a flexible bronchoscopy procedure on an intubated patient receiving mechanical ventilation?
    A. High peak inspiratory pressures
    B. Increase in tidal volume delivery
    C. Acute hypocapnia
    D. High minute ventilation alarm

FOOD FOR THOUGHT

As the field of respiratory therapy advances, the RT will be called on to assist in more complex respiratory procedures. Many procedures directly affect the respiratory system and should be within our area of expertise. This means you need to be constantly studying and always willing to learn new and exciting things. Remember, you need to be the lung expert!

23 Nutrition Assessment

WORD WIZARD

The language in Chapter 23 may read like a French menu—incomprehensibly. You may need to look up some of these terms before you can match them with their definitions.

Terms	Definitions
1. _____ Anergy	A. Excess nitrogenous waste in the blood.
2. _____ Anthropometrics	B. Relationship of weight to height.
3. _____ Azotemia	C. So thin that ribs stick out in persistent malnutrition.
4. _____ Basal metabolic rate	D. Energy measurement based on O_2 consumption and CO_2 production.
5. _____ Body mass index	E. Impaired immune response.
6. _____ Indirect calorimetry	F. Body measurements; the most frequently used are height and weight.
7. _____ Cachexic	G. Hourly resting energy consumption after fasting.

MEET THE OBJECTIVES

8. Describe the "most helpful" technique for nutrition assessment dietitians perform in the acute care setting.

9. What does BMI stand for, and what two variables are used to calculate it?

   A. BMI = _____

   B. Variable 1: _____

   C. Variable 2: _____

10. State the range of normal for BMI. (What is *your* BMI? What about your loved ones?)

11. State the formula for calculating ideal body weight.

    A. Males: _____

    B. Females: _____

    C. Calculate your own ideal body weight:

BIOCHEMICAL INDICATORS

12. Describe why serum proteins are useful as biochemical indicators when assessing nutritional status.

13. Why is monitoring albumin of limited use in assessing effectiveness of nutrition in the critical care setting?

14. What is the most commonly used biomarker for inflammation? What causes this biomarker to increase?

MACRONUTRIENTS

15. Name the three macronutrients that supply the body's energy requirements. State the kilocalories per gram for each.

	MACRONUTRIENT	KILOCALORIES PER GRAM
A.		
B.		
C.		

16. What percentage of patients with acute respiratory failure suffers from malnutrition?

17. List two reasons malnourished patients are difficult to wean from the ventilator.

    A. _____

    B. _____

18. Why are COPD patients often malnourished?

19. What are the consequences of malnutrition for respiratory muscles and response to hypoxia and hypercapnia?

INDIRECT CALORIMETRY

20. List three conditions where indirect calorimetry may be indicated.

    A. _____
    B. _____
    C. _____

21. What are the contraindications to indirect calorimetry in mechanically ventilated patients?

22. According to the AARC Clinical Practice Guidelines, closed-circuit calorimeters may reduce alveolar volume or increase work of breathing. Explain how these two hazards occur.

23. What actions should be taken to prepare a patient for indirect calorimetry?

A. 4 hours before the test: _____

B. 2 hours before the test: _____

C. 1 hour before the test: _____

24. Describe the most significant problem in performing indirect calorimetry on mechanically ventilated patients.

25. Interpret the following RQs and identify the general nutritional strategy.

	VALUE	INTERPRETATION	STRATEGY
A.	> 1		
B.	0.9 to 1		
C.	0.7 to 0.8		

26. State the formula for calculating REE using a pulmonary artery catheter.

27. What factors are used to adjust predicted REEs in patients? Give one example. (Go to Table 21-5.)

RESPIRATORY CONSEQUENCES

28. COPD patients have special dietary problems. Identify four factors that lead to poor intake in these patients.

A. _____

B. _____

C. _____

D. _____

29. What is the effect of high-carbohydrate loads on COPD patients?

30. What do the terms "enteral" and "parenteral" mean?

    A. Enteral: _____

    B. Parenteral: _____

31. How would the respiratory therapist confirm suspected aspiration of tube feedings? How is this complication avoided?

    A. Confirmation: _____

    B. Prevention: _____

    _____

    _____

32. Explain what happens when patients receive too much of the following substrates. Give a pulmonary example, please.

    A. Protein: _____

    B. Carbohydrates: _____

    C. Fat: _____

Pulmonary Pathologies

33. In general, COPD patients eat to optimize nutrition.

    A. How often? _____

    B. Calories? _____

34. People with asthma may greatly benefit from what specific type of fatty acids?

35. In addition to a lot of calories, what supplements do CF patients need?

SUMMARY CHECKLIST

Complete the following sentences by writing in the correct term(s) in the spaces provided.

36. The _____-_____ estimate daily resting energy expenditure.

37. _____ is a state of impaired metabolism in which the intake of nutrients falls short of the body's needs.

38. For patients with pulmonary disease, high _____ loads can increase carbon dioxide production.

39. Whenever possible, the _____ route should be used for supplying nutrients.

40. The likelihood of _____ during tube feedings can be minimized by _____ the head of the bed by _____.

CASE STUDY

A thin, undernourished COPD patient tells you that he has difficulty eating because he gets tired and short of breath during meals. Besides, food just doesn't taste as good now.

41. What eating pattern should be emphasized to this patient?

42. Make some suggestions that would increase his nutrient intake.

43. What other big problem might interfere with the patient's appetite?

WHAT DOES THE NBRC SAY?

44. A respiratory therapist is caring for a 66-year-old male patient with acute exacerbation of COPD. The therapist notes the patient is extremely thin, with ribs obviously showing on his chest. What term should the therapist use to document the patient's appearance?
    A. Malnourished
    B. Cyanotic
    C. Cachexic
    D. Wasted

45. Cystic fibrosis patients may need what dietary supplement to be able to absorb nutrients?
    A. Calcium
    B. Amino acids
    C. Enzymes
    D. Vitamin C

46. A patient with COPD is being counseled in a pulmonary rehabilitation program. What general nutrition recommendation would you give this individual?
    A. Eat frequent small meals.
    B. Restrict sodium intake.
    C. Restrict carbohydrate intake.
    D. Increase whole grain and fiber intake.

FOOD FOR THOUGHT

47. What type of nutritional strategy may help in weaning COPD patients from the ventilator?

24 Pulmonary Infections

WORD WIZARD

Write out the definition for each acronym.

CAP _____

HCAP _____

HAP _____

VAP _____

OK, now put the correct descriptive acronym next to these statements:

This patient got sick at home. _____

This patient got sick while receiving mechanical ventilation. _____

This patient got sick in the hospital. _____

This patient got sick in a nursing home. _____

CLASSIFICATION AND PATHOGENESIS

1. Define the term "empirical therapy."

2. The textbook definition of nosocomial pneumonia is now subdivided into HAP and VAP. Please describe these new terms *in depth* using the textbook criteria, because they are critical to your understanding of this life-threatening illness.
   A. HAP

   B. VAP

149

3. How common is lower respiratory tract infection (LRTI), and what are the estimated costs and mortality?

A. Prevalence: _____

_____

B. Costs: _____

_____

C. Mortality: _____

_____

4. List two patient populations that are at special risk for fatal forms of nosocomial pneumonia.

A. _____

B. _____

5. List four diseases acquired via inhalation of infectious particles.

A. _____

B. _____

C. _____

D. _____

6. List four of the patient populations at risk for aspiration of large volumes of gastric fluids.

A. _____

B. _____

C. _____

D. _____

7. State the two novel strategies mentioned in the book to reduce HAP or VAP in ventilated patients.

A. _____

B. _____

8. Describe the role of suctioning as a cause of lower respiratory tract inoculation.

9. Give the prime example of reactivation of a latent infection.

10. Why is it so important to know which organisms are commonly associated with pneumonia?

11. Which organism is most commonly identified as the cause of community-acquired pneumonia?

12. List the three most common atypical pathogens.

   A. _____

   B. _____

   C. _____

13. Why is no microbiologic identification made in 50% of pneumonia cases?

14. Name two viruses associated with pneumonia. What time of year are they encountered?
    A. Viruses:

      1. _____

      2. _____

    B. Time of year: _____

CLINICAL MANIFESTATIONS

15. In addition to fever, list the three respiratory symptoms patients with community-acquired pneumonia typically exhibit.

   A. _____

   B. _____

   C. _____

16. What is the classic, typical presentation of community-acquired pneumonia?

17. In intubated patients, VAP usually exhibits what three changes in the patient's condition?

A. _____

B. _____

C. _____

18. Describe the common radiograph abnormalities associated with pneumonia.

19. Why is the chest film of limited use in diagnosing pneumonia in critically ill patients?

RISK FACTORS

20. A number of factors predispose hospital patients to pneumonia, such as poor host defenses from underlying illness. Name five such "comorbidities."

A. _____

B. _____

C. _____

D. _____

E. _____

21. List four factors that expose the lungs to large numbers of microorganisms.

A. _____

B. _____

C. _____

D. _____

DIAGNOSTIC STUDIES

22. Why is determining the predominant causative organism via sputum Gram stain, culture, and sensitivity so useful in pneumonia patients?

23. Describe the process for collecting a good specimen by expectoration.

24. Describe the satisfactory specimen. (This is board examination material!)

25. Name the organism identified by each of the following specialized tests.

	TEST	ORGANISM
A.	Acid-fast stain	
B.	Direct fluorescent stain	
C.	Toluidine blue	
D.	Potassium hydroxide	

26. When should fiberoptic bronchoscopy be recommended in cases of community-acquired pneumonia?

27. List four techniques useful in confirming the diagnosis of nosocomial pneumonia.

A. _____

B. _____

C. _____

D. _____

28. Direct visualization of the lower airway is helpful in diagnosing VAP. What are the three criteria?

A. _____

B. _____

C. _____

29. What do the initials BAL stand for? Describe BAL.

A. BAL = _____

B. Description: _____

_____

_____

30. What is mini-BAL, and which health care professional performs the procedure?

THERAPY

31. What is the primary medical treatment for pneumonia?

32. How long is a typical course of treatment for pneumonia?

33. How long does it take for the radiograph to show resolution of pneumonia in young individuals? What about older patients?

A. Young patients: _____

B. Older patients: _____

PREVENTION

34. Immunization is one of the primary strategies for preventing community-acquired pneumonia. Individuals are immunized against which two organisms?

A. _____

B. _____

35. Identify three groups that should be immunized.

A. _____

B. _____

C. _____

36. Identify the three "probably effective" strategies for the prevention of nosocomial pneumonia.

A. _____

B. _____

C. _____

37. What positioning technique is useful in preventing pneumonia in patients?

38. What is the current medication for gastrointestinal bleeding prophylaxis that may be effective in preventing pneumonia?

CASE STUDIES

Case 1

A 55-year-old man arrives at the emergency department complaining of chills, fever, and chest pain on inspiration. He is coughing up rusty-colored sputum. He admits to a history of heavy smoking and regular use of alcoholic beverages. Physical examination reveals a heart rate of 125 beats/min, respiratory rate of 30 breaths/min, and temperature of 104° F. He has inspiratory crackles in the right lower lobe. Blood gases reveal a pH of 7.34, $PaCO_2$ of 50 mm Hg, and PaO_2 of 58 mm Hg.

39. What is the most likely diagnosis? Support your answer based on the clinical signs and symptoms.

40. What immediate treatment should you initiate?

41. Give at least five reasons the patient is at risk of dying from his condition.

   A. _____

   B. _____

   C. _____

   D. _____

   E. _____

Case 2

A patient is intubated and on the ventilator following a head injury. On the third day following his craniotomy, he develops a fever. During routine suctioning, you notice his secretions are thick and yellow. Breath sounds are decreased in the left lower lobe.

42. What is the role of the artificial airway in development of pneumonia?

43. What test would you recommend at this time to help confirm a diagnosis?

WHAT DOES THE NBRC SAY?

44. A patient is seen in the ED with fever, chills, and tachypnea. He states he feels weak and short of breath. The vitals are T 101.4° F, f 28, HR 121, BP 140/96, and SpO_2 88% on room air. What should the respiratory therapist do first?
    A. Obtain a sputum specimen.
    B. Request a chest x-ray.
    C. Place the patient on antibiotics.
    D. Place the patient on oxygen.

45. A 14-year-old is admitted to the medical floor with "acute exacerbation of asthma secondary to lung infection." While administering bronchodilator therapy, the respiratory therapist observes the patient producing moderate amounts of thick yellow phlegm. What should the therapist recommend at this point?
    A. Obtain a sputum specimen.
    B. Request a chest x-ray.
    C. Place the patient on antibiotics.
    D. Place the patient on oxygen.

46. The gold standard for confirming diagnosis of pneumonia in an acutely ill patient is
    A. sputum culture.
    B. chest x-ray.
    C. blood cultures.
    D. CT scan.

47. A person with AIDS presents in the ED with profound hypoxemia, shortness of breath, and nonproductive cough. Physical examination findings suggest bilateral lower lobe pneumonia. Which of the following organisms is most likely to be seen in this particular individual?
    1. *Pneumocystis jiroveci*
    2. *Streptococcus pneumoniae*
    3. *Mycobacterium tuberculosis*
        A. 1 only
        B. 2 and 3 only
        C. 1 and 3 only
        D. 1, 2, and 3

48. New onset of fever accompanied by purulent secretions and a new infiltrate on the chest film in an intubated patient are strongly suggestive of
    A. VAP.
    B. HAP.
    C. CAP.
    D. HCAP.

49. The respiratory therapist suspects that one of her ventilator patients is at high risk for developing pneumonia. What general action should the therapist take?
    A. Request a chest x-ray.
    B. Elevate the head of the bed.
    C. Implement the VAP protocol.
    D. Implement an in-line suction catheter.

FOOD FOR THOUGHT

50. What is the role of the RT in educating at-risk populations about methods to prevent pneumonia?

25 Obstructive Lung Disease: Chronic Obstructive Pulmonary Disease (COPD), Asthma, and Related Diseases

CHRONIC OBSTRUCTIVE PULMONARY DISEASE

1. *Chronic obstructive pulmonary disease* is defined by the American Thoracic Society (ATS) by four key concepts. Please elaborate on the following.

   A. Limitation: _____

   B. Progressive: _____

   C. Inflammatory: _____

   D. Systemic: _____

2. According to the National Health and Nutrition Examination Survey (NHANES) data, what percentage of the U.S. population has mild *or* moderate COPD?

   Mild: _____

   Moderate: _____

3. How does COPD rank as a leading cause of death in the United States, and why is this condition strikingly different from heart disease or stroke?

RISK FACTORS AND PATHOPHYSIOLOGY

4. It is estimated 80% to 90% of cigarette smokers get COPD. What is the other major cause of emphysema?

5. Briefly explain the protease-antiprotease hypothesis of emphysema.

6. Describe three mechanisms of airflow obstruction in COPD.

A. _____

B. _____

C. _____

CLINICAL SIGNS

7. List four common symptoms of COPD.

A. _____

B. _____

C. _____

D. _____

8. Compare the onset of dyspnea in typical cases of COPD with that of α_1-antitrypsin deficiency.

9. What physical change in the chest wall occurs as a result of prolonged hyperinflation?

10. List three other late signs of COPD.

A. _____

B. _____

C. _____

11. Compare chronic bronchitis, emphysema, and α_1-antitrypsin deficiency in terms of the following features.

	FEATURES	CHRONIC BRONCHITIS	EMPHYSEMA	α_1-ANTITRYPSIN DEFICIENCY
A.	Age of onset			
B.	Family history			
C.	Smoker			
D.	Lung volume			
E.	D_{LCO}			
F.	FEV_1/FVC			
G.	Radiograph			

Management

12. Why would it be important to differentiate asthma from other forms of COPD? List some distinguishing characteristics of each.

   A. Why differentiate?

   B. Features characteristic of COPD:

   C. Features characteristic of asthma:

13. Reversible airflow obstruction is defined as an increase of what amount?

   A. Percentage: _____

   B. Milliliters: _____

14. Why is bronchodilator therapy recommended for COPD? What types of drugs are used?

   A. Why? _____

   B. Types of drugs? _____

15. Discuss the role of inhaled steroids (ICS) in COPD. Which group should receive ICS according to the GOLD guidelines/ATS guidelines?

16. List the four important elements of managing an acute exacerbation of COPD due to purulent bronchitis.

A. _____

B. _____

C. _____

D. _____

17. When hypercapnia and respiratory failure are present (and pH is < 7.3), what patient characteristics are present in a good candidate for noninvasive ventilation?

18. What is the primary goal of pulmonary rehabilitation?

19. A comprehensive smoking cessation program usually includes what three elements?

A. _____

B. _____

C. _____

20. Three treatments for COPD have been shown to prolong survival. Please elaborate.
A. Oxygen:

B. Quitting smoking:

C. Lung volume reduction surgery (LVRS):

21. What is the relationship between bronchodilator therapy and home oxygen therapy?

22. You need to know the indications for continuous oxygen. Please give the correct values for

A. Resting PaO$_2$: _____

B. Hematocrit: _____

C. ECG: _____

ASTHMA

Overview

23. What is the difference between older definitions and the more current view of asthma?

24. What percentage of people in the United States is believed to have asthma? (In 2002, it was estimated to be 5%!)

Etiology and Pathogenesis

25. Airway inflammation and bronchial hyperreactivity result in airflow obstruction. List four triggers:

A. _____

B. _____

C. _____

D. _____

26. What happens when a patient with asthma inhales an allergen to which he or she is sensitized?

27. Describe early and late asthmatic reactions (EAR and LAR, respectively).

   A. EAR:

   B. LAR:

Clinical Signs

28. What factor plays a key role in suggesting and establishing a diagnosis of asthma?

29. List four classic symptoms of asthma.

   A. _____

   B. _____

   C. _____

   D. _____

30. List five conditions that can mimic the wheezing of asthma.

   A. _____

   B. _____

   C. _____

   D. _____

   E. _____

31. Bronchial provocation is the specialized test used to demonstrate obstruction in patients with suspected asthma who are symptom-free at the time of testing. Name the drug used for this test and what response indicates hyperresponsiveness.

   A. Drug: _____

   B. Response: _____

Management

32. Explain control of asthma in terms of the following criteria:

A. Symptoms: _____

_____

B. β_2-agonists: _____

_____

C. Exercise: _____

_____

D. PEFR/FEV$_1$: _____

_____

E. Exacerbations: _____

_____

33. Give the criteria and actions for green, yellow, and red peak flow zones.

	ZONE	PEFR % PREDICTED	TREATMENT/ACTION
A.	Green		
B.	Yellow		
C.	Red		

34. Compare the use of inhaled corticosteroids and bronchodilators in treating asthma.

35. Name the two common side effects of inhaled steroids and two ways to control them.

A. _____

B. _____

C. Control/reduce side effects:

1. _____

2. _____

36. Leukotriene modifiers such as montelukast sodium (Singulair) are popular and useful for which categories of asthma? Do these drugs replace steroids?

37. What type of drug is the first-line treatment for all types of acute bronchospasm?

38. What is the benefit of using anticholinergics such as ipratropium in the day-to-day management of asthma?

39. List three factors you should monitor in a patient hospitalized with acute asthma.

    A. _____

    B. _____

    C. _____

40. Management of asthma should be aggressive, including two specific types of medications along with oxygen. Discuss the use of β-agonists and steroids in this specific situation.

    A. β-agonists: _____

    _____

    B. Steroids: _____

    _____

41. How can you prevent allergic reactions in patients with asthma through immunotherapy?

42. What is EIA? List two prophylactic drug treatments.

    A. EIA = _____

    B. Prophylaxis:

        1. _____

        2. _____

43. Define occupational asthma. What is the most common cause?

44. What is the only way to eliminate occupational asthma once an individual is sensitized?

45. What drug is particularly helpful in the treatment of cough-variant asthma?

46. List three medications that may be helpful in treating nocturnal asthma.

A. _____

B. _____

C. _____

47. What recommendations would you make to a patient who has aspirin sensitivity?

48. What is the effect of pregnancy on women with asthma?

49. Discuss the use of asthma medications during pregnancy.

50. GER (most of us call it GERD) can also play a role in asthma. Any ideas on how to help?

51. A surprising number of people with asthma have nose and sinus problems. What types of inhalers do they need?

BRONCHIECTASIS

52. What is the clinical hallmark of bronchiectasis?

53. What test is now considered definitive for diagnosing bronchiectasis?

54. List the three major anatomic patterns seen in bronchiectasis.

    A. _____

    B. _____

    C. _____

55. List the two primary treatments for bronchiectasis.

    A. _____

    B. _____

And if these don't work, the patient needs to have _____.

CASE STUDIES

Case 1

A 70-year-old man's chief complaint is dyspnea on exertion. He has a smoking history of two packs per day for the past 50 years. He has a barrel-shaped chest and significantly decreased breath sounds. His chest radiograph shows hyperinflation, especially in the apices, flattened diaphragms, and a small heart. He admits to a morning cough but denies significant sputum production.

56. What is the most likely diagnosis?

57. Calculate the patient's pack-years.

58. What factor should you focus on to help the patient control his condition?

A 60-year-old man has smoked a pack of cigarettes per day since he was a teenager. He complains of a chronic productive cough that is producing thick, yellow sputum. He is admitted to the medical floor with a fever and shortness of breath. Blood gases reveal pH of 7.35, $PaCO_2$ of 50 mm Hg, and PaO_2 of 57 mm Hg. Physical examination shows pedal edema, distended neck veins, and use of accessory muscles of ventilation. He has scattered wheezing and rhonchi on auscultation.

59. What type of COPD is most likely in this case?

60. What should you do with his sputum the next time he coughs productively?

61. What is the immediate respiratory treatment in this case?

62. What respiratory medications would you recommend?

A 44-year-old man complains of dyspnea on exertion. He is a nonsmoker but drinks wine with his meals. He has a barrel-shaped chest and very decreased breath sounds. His chest radiograph shows hyperinflation, especially in the bases. History reveals that his father and uncle both died of "lung problems."

63. What is the most likely cause of the patient's COPD symptoms? Justify your answer based on the information presented.

Chapter **25** Obstructive Lung Disease

64. What treatments are available for this condition?

A 15-year-old boy complains that he cannot catch his breath when he exercises. He states that he coughs a lot, especially in the winter. His breath sounds are clear, and his physical examination is unremarkable.

65. What do you suspect is the problem?

66. How could a definitive diagnosis be made?

WHAT DOES THE NBRC SAY?

Use the following data to answer questions 67 through 72.

A 20-year-old woman who has a history of asthma is brought to the emergency department in respiratory distress. Your assessment of the patient reveals the following:

pH	7.47
$PaCO_2$	33 mm Hg
PaO_2	72 mm Hg
HCO_3^-	23 mEq/L
RR	28
HR	115
PEFR	200 L/min

67. Which of the following breath sounds would you expect to hear in this patient?
   A. Inspiratory crackles
   B. Expiratory wheezing
   C. Inspiratory stridor
   D. Expiratory rhonchi

68. The arterial blood gas results indicate the presence of
   A. acute respiratory alkalosis.
   B. acute metabolic alkalosis.
   C. chronic respiratory acidosis.
   D. acute respiratory acidosis.

69. You are asked to initiate oxygen therapy. What would you recommend?
    A. Simple mask at 10 L/min
    B. Nonrebreathing mask at 15 L/min
    C. Nasal cannula at 2 L/min
    D. Air-entrainment mask at 0.50 F_IO_2

70. What therapy would you recommend after the oxygen is in place?
    A. 2 puffs ipratropium (Atrovent) via MDI
    B. 2.5 mg albuterol (Proventil) via SVN
    C. Intravenous theophylline administration
    D. Intravenous antibiotics

71. Blood gases are repeated 30 minutes after the oxygen therapy is initiated.
pH	7.42
$PaCO_2$	38 mm Hg
PaO_2	86 mm Hg
HCO_3^-	23 mEq/L
RR	24
HR	88
PEFR	210 L/min

    Which of the following has shown significant improvement based on this information?
    A. Compliance
    B. Resistance
    C. Oxygenation
    D. Ventilation

72. Intravenous steroids and repeated bronchodilators have been given. The patient is now receiving F_IO_2 of 0.40.
pH	7.34
$PaCO_2$	53 mm Hg
PaO_2	74 mm Hg
HCO_3^-	26 mEq/L
RR	18
HR	125
PEFR	110 L/min

    What would you suggest at this point?
    A. Increase FiO_2 to 0.50
    B. Continuous nebulization of bronchodilators
    C. Administration of intravenous bicarbonate
    D. Intubation and mechanical ventilation

73. A patient with COPD and CO_2 retention is admitted for an acute exacerbation of her disease. The physician requests your suggestion for initiating oxygen therapy. Which of the following would you recommend?
    A. Nasal cannula at 6 L/min
    B. Air-entrainment mask at 28%
    C. Simple mask at 2 L/min
    D. Partial rebreathing mask at 8 L/min

74. A PFT on a 65-year-old woman indicates airflow obstruction with mild air-trapping. The patient is coughing up thick sputum. Which of the following diagnoses is most likely?
    A. Cystic fibrosis
    B. Pneumonia
    C. Pulmonary fibrosis
    D. Bronchiectasis

75. A PFT on a 56-year-old man with a history of smoking shows increased TLC and RV. The D_{LCO} is reduced. What diagnosis is suggested by these findings?
    A. Emphysema
    B. Pneumonia
    C. Sarcoidosis
    D. Pneumoconiosis

76. Spirometry is performed before and after bronchodilator administration. Which of the following indicates a therapeutic response?
    1. FEV_1 increased by 10%.
    2. FVC increased by 300 ml.
    3. PEFR increased by 5%.
       A. 1 only
       B. 2 only
       C. 1 and 2 only
       D. 1 and 3 only

FOOD FOR THOUGHT

77. Because only 15% of smokers actually show big declines in airflow, why should we encourage all patients to quit smoking?

78. What is omalizumab (Xolair), and how does it work for asthma?

26 Interstitial Lung Disease

WORD WIZARD

Match the correct definition with the correct term.

Definitions	Terms
1. _____ Asbestosis	A. Formation of scar tissue in the lung without known cause
2. _____ Corticosteroids	B. Respiratory disorder characterized by fibrotic infiltrates in the lower lobes
3. _____ Drug-related lung disease	C. Inflammatory reaction provoked by inhalation of organic dusts
4. _____ Lymphangioleiomyomatosis	D. Lung disease caused by chemotherapy agents, for example
5. _____ Hypersensitivity pneumonitis	E. Asbestosis, chronic silicosis, and coal workers' pneumoconiosis
6. _____ Idiopathic pulmonary fibrosis	F. Restrictive disorder associated with pleural abnormalities and lung tumors
7. _____ Interstitial lung disease	G. Disorder of unknown origin that results in formation of epithelioid tubercles
8. _____ Interstitium	H. Hormones associated with control of body processes
9. _____ Occupational ILD	I. A rare disorder of abnormal smooth muscle tissue proliferating around small airways leading to severe obstruction and destruction of alveoli with resultant thin-walled cyst formation
10. _____ Organizing pneumonitis	J. The area between the capillaries and the alveolar space
11. _____ Pulmonary Langerhans cell histiocytosis	K. The revised term for *bronchiolitis obliterans organizing pneumonia*
12. _____ Sarcoidosis	L. Disorder caused by long-term exposure to sand and stone dust
13. _____ Silicosis	M. Nodules are star-shaped and destroy adjacent lung tissue

CLINICAL SIGNS AND SYMPTOMS OF ILD

14. Patients with interstitial lung disease (ILD) of many different etiologies will usually present with which two common complaints?

   A. _____

   B. _____

15. Describe the breath sounds typically heard in ILD.

16. List the late signs of ILD.

17. Physical signs of underlying connective tissue disease include what three features?

A. _____

B. _____

C. _____

18. Describe the classic and late radiographic findings in idiopathic pulmonary fibrosis; use the colorful descriptive terms from *Egan's*. What are the late-stage findings?

A. Classic: _____

B. Late: _____

19. Discuss the effects of ILD on the following pulmonary function variables.

	VARIABLE	EFFECT OF ILD
A.	FEV_1	
B.	FVC	
C.	FEV_1/FVC	
D.	D_{LCO}	
E.	Lung volumes	
F.	Compliance	

SPECIFIC TYPES OF ILD

20. List the three most common types of occupational ILD.

A. _____

B. _____

C. _____

21. What do these examples have in common?

22. Why is pulmonary involvement in connective tissue disorders often undetected until late in the course of the disease?

23. List three common connective disorders associated with lung disease.

A. _____

B. _____

C. _____

24. What is the name for chronic exposure to inhaled organic material that results in progressive scarring of the lung?

25. What factor is critical to identifying the cause of this condition?

26. What is meant by the term "idiopathic"?

27. Let's compare the two idiopathic lung diseases discussed in the text.

		Idiopathic Pulmonary Fibrosis (IPF)	Sarcoidosis
A.	Age		
B.	Symptoms		
C.	Treatment		
D.	Prognosis		

28. Discuss the common areas of treatment for hypersensitivity pneumonitis and occupational lung disease.

29. What is the primary drug therapy for ILD?

30. What is the most common respiratory therapy modality for ILD?

31. What is the only therapy shown to prolong life in end-stage ILD?

A 48-year-old man is admitted for dyspnea on exertion and a dry cough of unknown origin. The chest radiograph shows bilateral reticulonodular infiltrates. Pulse oximetry indicates mild hypoxemia on room air. History reveals that the patient is a hay farmer.

32. What is the most likely diagnosis?

33. What is the most likely cause of the lung disease? What are some other possible causes?

Case 2

A retired Pearl Harbor shipyard worker states that he has had a cough for some time but recently began expectorating some blood. He has bibasilar inspiratory crackles, with otherwise clear breath sounds. A chest radiograph shows reticulonodular infiltrates in both lower lobes. The radiologist also notes the presence of a small right-sided pleural effusion and the presence of pleural plaques and pleural fibrosis. PFTs reveal a normal FEV_1 %, decreased TLC and RV, and a decreased D_{LCO}.

34. What is the most likely pulmonary diagnosis?

35. What other information would be helpful in making a determination?

36. What type of disorder is suggested by the PFT results?

37. A patient with a history of sarcoidosis presents in the emergency department with shortness of breath. Vital signs are T 99, P 114, f 32, BP 138/88 and SpO_2 82%. The respiratory care practitioner would
    A. administer oxygen via nasal cannula at 2 L/min.
    B. request a STAT portable AP chest x-ray.
    C. perform a STAT ABG.
    D. administer albuterol.

FOOD FOR THOUGHT

38. What is the general term for all lung diseases that cause a reduction in lung volumes without a reduction in flow

    rates?

27 Pleural Diseases

Chapter 27 introduces lots of important new terms. Match these pleural puzzlers to their definitions.

Terms	Definitions
1. _____ Bronchopleural fistula	A. Pleural effusion high in protein
2. _____ Chylothorax	B. Air leak from the lung to the pleural space
3. _____ Empyema	C. Membrane covering the surface of the chest wall
4. _____ Exudative effusion	D. Pleural fluid rich with triglycerides from a ruptured thoracic duct
5. _____ Hemothorax	E. Pleural pain
6. _____ Parietal pleura	F. Pus-filled pleural effusion
7. _____ Pleural effusion	G. Blood in the pleural space
8. _____ Pleurisy	H. Abnormal collection of fluid in the pleural space
9. _____ Pleurodesis	I. Pneumothorax without underlying lung disease
10. _____ Pneumothorax	J. Air under pressure in the pleural space
11. _____ Primary spontaneous pneumothorax	K. Procedure that fuses the pleura to prevent pneumothorax
12. _____ Reexpansion pulmonary edema	L. Air in the pleural space
13. _____ Secondary spontaneous pneumothorax	M. Occurs when the lung is rapidly inflated after compression by pleural fluid
14. _____ Tension pneumothorax	N. Pneumothorax that occurs with underlying lung disease
15. _____ Thoracentesis	O. Low-protein effusion caused by CHF or cirrhosis
16. _____ Transudative pleural effusion	P. Chest wall puncture for diagnostic or therapeutic purposes
17. _____ Visceral pleura	Q. Membrane that lines the lung surface

THE PLEURAL SPACE

18. How are the pleura of the American buffalo different from those of humans? What is the clinical significance for the buffalo, and when are humans in the same situation?

19. Describe both the visceral and parietal pleura. Where do the two meet and become a single, continuous pleural membrane?

20. Is normal intrapleural pressure positive or negative, and what effect does this have on fluid movement?

21. Explain why pleural pressures are different at the apex and lung bases.

PLEURAL EFFUSIONS

22. Give a brief explanation of how each of the following conditions can cause transudative pleural effusions.
    A. CHF:

    B. Hypoalbuminemia:

C. Liver disease:

D. Lymph obstruction:

E. CVP line:

23. What is the most common cause of clinical pleural effusions?

24. What is the general cause of exudative pleural effusions?

25. Give a brief explanation of the cause of these exudative pleural effusions.
    A. Parapneumonic

    B. Malignant

C. Chylothorax

D. Hemothorax

26. What change in pulmonary function is associated with pleural effusion?

27. In what specific portion of the upright chest film is pleural effusion visualized?

28. Describe the specific type of chest film used to improve visualization of pleural effusions.

29. What type of imaging is the most sensitive test for identification of pleural effusions?

30. List the three major risks of thoracentesis.

    A. _____

    B. _____

    C. _____

31. Identify the purpose of each of the chambers in the three-bottle chest tube drainage system shown on the next page.

    A. _____

    B. _____

    C. _____

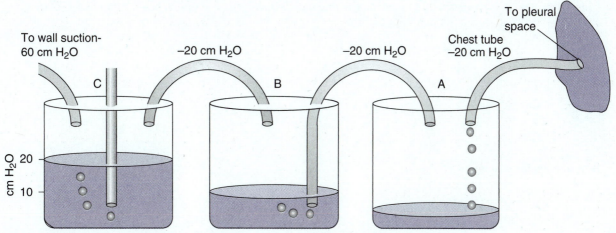

To wall suction-
60 cm H_2O

To pleural space

Chest tube
-20 cm H_2O

-20 cm H_2O

-20 cm H_2O

C

B

A

cm H_2O

20

10

The standard three-bottle system is the basis for all commercial chest tube drainage systems.

PNEUMOTHORAX

32. List two symptoms that are common to almost all cases of pneumothorax.

    A. _____

    B. _____

33. What is the most common type of traumatic pneumothorax, and how is it treated? Give three examples.

34. Compare blunt and penetrating chest trauma as causes of pneumothorax. How does treatment differ in these two situations?

35. What special technique may be helpful to visualize pneumothorax in a newborn?

36. Compare the two major types of spontaneous pneumothorax.

37. Tension pneumothorax can be a life-threatening medical emergency. It is a common board exam item. Please give short clear explanations for items A through D.

A. Definition

B. Radiographic finding

C. Clinical signs

D. Treatment

38. Compare the outcomes of early clinical diagnosis and treatment of tension pneumothorax with delayed diagnosis.

39. How does oxygen administration assist in resolution of a pneumothorax?

40. What is BPF? How does mechanical ventilation perpetuate this problem? What special modes of ventilation may be indicated?

A. BPF = _____

B. Ventilators perpetuate BPF by: _____

C. Adjust ventilator for BPF patient by: _____

CASE STUDIES

Case 1

A mathematics instructor with a history of CHF is admitted with a complaint of pain on inspiration. Her respirations are rapid and shallow, and her heart rate is 104 beats/min. The pulse oximeter shows a saturation of 93% on room air. Breath sounds are very decreased on the right side, with crackles in the left base. Chest wall movement is markedly less on the right. The chest radiograph shows opacification of the right lung, with shift of mediastinal structures to the left. Diagnostic percussion reveals a dull note on the right side.

41. What do you think is wrong with this patient's right lung? Support your conclusion with at least five pieces of information from the case.

A. I think the patient has a _____ because

1. _____

2. _____

3. _____

4. _____

5. _____

42. What would you recommend as the first respiratory intervention?

43. How could this disorder be resolved?

A tall, thin young male respiratory care instructor is admitted with a complaint of pain on inspiration. His respirations are rapid and shallow, and his heart rate is 104 beats/min. The pulse oximeter shows a saturation of 93% on room air. Breath sounds are very decreased on the right side, and clear in the left base. Chest wall movement is markedly less on the right. The chest radiograph shows a dark area without lung markings on the right side, with a shift of mediastinal structures to the left. Diagnostic percussion reveals increased resonance on the right side.

44. What do you think is wrong with this patient's right lung? Support your conclusion with at least five pieces of information from the case.

    A. I think this patient has a _____ because

      1. _____

      2. _____

      3. _____

      4. _____

      5. _____

45. What would you recommend as the first respiratory intervention?

46. How could this disorder be resolved?

WHAT DOES THE NBRC SAY?

Circle the best answer.

47. Immediately after insertion of a central line via the subclavian vein, an intubated patient becomes dyspneic. The respiratory therapist should recommend which of the following diagnostic tests?
A. 12-lead ECG
B. Chest radiograph
C. ABG
D. Bedside spirometry

48. The middle bottle of a three-bottle chest drainage system is used as a _____.
    A. water seal
    B. fluid collection
    C. means of applying vacuum to the chest
    D. measurement of improvement of the pneumothorax

49. A chest tube is placed anteriorly between the second and third ribs. The tube is probably intended to treat a
    A. chylothorax.
    B. hemothorax.
    C. transudative pleural effusion.
    D. pneumothorax.

50. A patient is suspected of having a pleural effusion. Which x-ray position is most appropriate to confirm this diagnosis?
    A. AP chest film
    B. Lateral decubitus chest film
    C. Apical lordotic chest film
    D. PA chest film

51. Thoracentesis is performed and 1500 ml of fluid is removed from the right chest. Which of the following is likely to occur as a result?
    A. Pulmonary edema in the right lung
    B. Stridor and respiratory distress
    C. Pneumothorax in the right lung
    D. Atelectasis in the right lung

52. All of the following would be useful in differentiating right mainstem intubation from left-sided pneumothorax *except*
    A. chest radiograph.
    B. diagnostic percussion.
    C. auscultation.
    D. lung compliance measurement.

53. Following an IPPB treatment, a COPD patient complains of sudden severe chest pain. What is the respiratory therapist's first priority in this situation?
    A. Notify the physician of the problem.
    B. Initiate oxygen therapy.
    C. Recommend a chest radiograph.
    D. Perform an arterial blood gas.

54. A patient develops subcutaneous emphysema following a motor vehicle accident involving multiple rib fractures. What action should the respiratory therapist take in this situation?
    A. Perform bedside spirometry.
    B. Initiate oxygen therapy.
    C. Recommend a chest radiograph.
    D. Perform an arterial blood gas.

FOOD FOR THOUGHT

55. What is meant by the term "ascites"? Besides causing effusions, how could ascites affect respiratory function?

56. How is thoracentesis modified to prevent reexpansion pulmonary edema?

57. What is subcutaneous emphysema, and what relationship does it have to pneumothorax?

28 Pulmonary Vascular Disease

Complete the following paragraph by writing in the correct terms in the spaces provided.

When the pressure inside the lung vessels is elevated, a condition called pulmonary _____ exists. Prolonged

bed rest could result in formation of a venous _____. Most clots form in the _____ veins of the

lower legs. The blood clot could travel to the lung where it is called a pulmonary _____, or PE. If this process

results in death of the lung tissue, it is called pulmonary _____. Small particles of fat or air could also form
an embolus. Chronic elevation of pulmonary blood pressure will eventually cause a form of right heart failure known

as cor _____.

MEET THE OBJECTIVES

1. How many people develop thromboembolic disease each year in the United States?

2. How do these clots form? Where are they most likely to form first?

   Which patient population or situations have the most risk for this sort of pathology?

3. Explain how pulmonary embolism (PE) affects the heart and lungs as they try to function together. (Just give the basic idea.)

4. What is the primary hemodynamic consequence of PE?

5. List the two most common symptoms of PE.

    A. _____

    B. _____

6. List the three most frequent physical findings associated with PE.

    A. _____

    B. _____

    C. _____

7. List the two most common ECG abnormalities associated with PE.

    A. _____

    B. _____

8. How is the chest radiograph helpful in diagnosing pulmonary embolism?

9. How helpful are arterial blood gases (ABGs) in ruling out PE? What benefit does an ABG provide in these cases?

10. One rapid blood test has been developed to help rule out embolism. Why isn't D-dimer as good for some inpatients?

11. Which test is considered the "gold standard" for the diagnosis of DVT?

FINDING PE

12. Because of the high mortality rate, it is important to make a definitive diagnosis of pulmonary embolus. What two tests are reasonably sensitive and reliable in confirming this diagnosis?

    A. _____

    B. _____

13. What is the relationship of the ventilation ($\dot{V}$) and perfusion ($\dot{Q}$) portions of scans in making a high-probability diagnosis of PE?

14. Discuss advantages and disadvantages of helical CT scans for PE.
    A. Advantages:

    B. Disadvantages:

ASSESS AND TEST

15. Prophylaxis for DVT is either pharmacologic or mechanical. Give three examples of each.
    A. Pharmacologic prophylaxis

    1. _____

    2. _____

    3. _____

    B. Mechanical prophylaxis

    1. _____

    2. _____

    3. _____

16. What is the standard pharmacologic therapy for existing DVT or PE? What is the mechanism of action? What are the risks?

A. Drug:

_____

B. Action:

_____

C. Risks:

_____

17. How are thrombolytics different from anticoagulants? Can they be given together?

18. Give three examples of thrombolytic drugs.

A. _____

B. _____

C. _____

19. List the mechanical options available for treatment of massive PE.

20. When are vena cava filters indicated?

21. Define pulmonary hypertension.

22. Describe the epidemiology of IPH in terms of age, gender, symptoms, mortality, and genetic factors.

   A.   Age: _____

   B.   Gender: _____

   C.   Genetics: _____

   D.   Symptoms: _____

   E.   Mortality: _____

23. How is IPH diagnosed?

24. Why is it so important to provide oxygen as needed to keep up the patient's saturations in this condition?

25. Which drug treatment is given via inhalation?

26. Explain the role of alveolar hypoxia in the development of pulmonary hypertension.

27. What other factors seen in COPD contribute to this condition?

28. What is the only treatment that improves survival in patients with COPD and pulmonary hypertension? What treatments might help?

A 60-year-old man underwent total knee replacement. Two days after surgery, he complains of dyspnea and anxiety. Physical examination reveals a heart rate of 110, respiratory rate of 28, blood pressure of 115/80 mm Hg, and SpO_2 of 93% on room air. Breath sounds are clear except for faint inspiratory crackles in both bases.

29. Why is this patient at risk for PE?

30. What additional diagnostic tests would be helpful in ruling out other potential pulmonary problems?

31. What treatment would you provide as a respiratory therapist?

32. What medical treatment should be initiated if a diagnosis of PE is confirmed?

Circle the best answer.

33. A patient who is being mechanically ventilated shows an increased V_D/V_T ratio. Which of the following disorders could be responsible?
    A. Atelectasis
    B. Pneumonia
    C. Pulmonary embolism
    D. Pleural effusion

34. Which of the following is the most appropriate test to confirm the presence of a suspected PE?
    A. Chest radiograph
    B. Pulmonary angiography
    C. Bronchogram
    D. Arterial blood gas

35. A ventilation/perfusion scan reveals a defect in perfusion in the right lower lobe without a corresponding decrease in ventilation. Which of the following is the most probable diagnosis?
    A. Right lower lobe atelectasis
    B. Acute pulmonary embolus
    C. Pneumothorax
    D. Pneumonia

36. A patient presents in the ED with severe dyspnea and complains of chest pain. His respiratory rate is 24 and his minute volume is 14 L. ABG results show pH 7.44, $PaCO_2$ 37, and PaO_2 100. What is the most likely cause of a normal CO_2 when a patient has a large increase in minute ventilation?
    A. Acute myocardial infarction
    B. Spontaneous pneumothorax
    C. Pulmonary embolus
    D. Pneumonia

FOOD FOR THOUGHT

37. What is the most common cause of pulmonary hypertension worldwide?

38. Discuss the pros and cons of moving a critically ill ventilator patient to imaging for a $\dot{V}/\dot{Q}$ scan to confirm a suspected diagnosis of PE.

29 Acute Respiratory Distress Syndrome (ARDS)

WORD WIZARD

Write out the definitions of terminology found in Chapter 29.

1. ALI: _____

2. APRV: _____

3. ARDS: _____

4. CHF: _____

5. ECMO: _____

6. $ECCO_2R$: _____

7. GI tract: _____

8. HFV: _____

9. MODS: _____

10. PMNs: _____

11. PEEP: _____

MEET THE OBJECTIVES

General Considerations

12. For each of the following general categories, name two common conditions leading to hydrostatic pulmonary edema:

	CATEGORY	CONDITIONS
A.	Cardiac	1.
		2.
B.	Vascular	1.
		2.
C.	Volume overload	1.
		2.

13. List four primary and four secondary risk factors or "triggers" for ARDS.
   A. Primary (direct injury)

   1. _____

   2. _____

   3. _____

   4. _____

   B. Secondary (indirect injury)

   1. _____

   2. _____

   3. _____

   4. _____

14. Compare the recommended definitions for ARDS using the AECC criteria and the Berlin criteria.

	AECC Criteria (1994)	Berlin Criteria (2012)
Timing of onset		
Risk factor		
Exclusion of hydrostatic edema		
Hypoxemia		
Chest imaging		

15. What five areas must be addressed to prevent further lung injury in ARDS?

   A. _____

   B. _____

   C. _____

   D. _____

   E. _____

Ventilator Strategies

16. How does optimal PEEP differ from PEEP that delivers the best PaO_2? (The NBRC loves this one!)

17. We can attempt to avoid barotrauma by maintaining plateau pressures below what value?

18. PEEP should be adjusted to maintain what F_iO_2 and PaO_2?

19. What is the tidal volume range used in ARDS patients?

20. What is meant by "permissive hypercapnia"? What is the goal of this ventilator strategy?

21. In what condition is permissive hypercapnia contraindicated? Why?

Innovative Strategies

22. A man is 6 feet tall. He has ARDS. What is the formula? The IBW? The right volume?
    A. Formula:

    B. Calculate the IBW.

    C. What range of tidal volume do you have to work with according to ARDSNet?

23. What mode of mechanical ventilation is best for patients with ARDS to prevent against lung damage?

24. How can patient positioning be radically altered to improve gas exchange?

25. Both ECMO and ECCO$_2$R facilitate gas exchange via what type of device?

26. Exogenous surfactant is helpful in treating infant respiratory distress syndrome and when surfactant is washed out of the adult lung. What's the story on using this with ARDS in adults?

Pharmacologic Treatments

27. Surfactant is not currently recommended for ARDS. What patient group does respond to surfactant administration?

28. What was the potential role of nitric oxide (NO) in treating ARDS?

29. What is the consequence of sudden discontinuation of inhaled NO?

SUMMARY CHECKLIST

Complete the following sentences by filling in the correct term(s) in the blank(s) provided.

30. CHF and ARDS are common causes of acute _____ failure that have similar initial _____ presentations.

31. CHF-associated pulmonary edema is due to elevated _____ pressures in the _____.

32. ARDS-associated pulmonary edema results from _____ injury to the lungs.

33. Ventilator strategies for patients with ARDS are designed to minimize ventilator _____ lung _____ by using _____, low _____ volumes, reduced airway _____, and nontoxic levels of inspired _____.

Case 1

A 5-foot, 6-inch, 143-lb (65-kg) teenager did not listen when his mom told him not to pop his pimples. Now he is in the ICU with a temperature of 103° F, blood pressure of 80/50 mm Hg, heart rate of 120 beats/min, and SpO_2 of 88% on 100% oxygen. His pulmonary capillary wedge pressure is 14 mm Hg, and cardiac output is 8 L/min. Breath sounds reveal coarse crackles throughout the lungs. The patient is intubated and currently is being ventilated with a tidal volume of 800 ml, frequency of 14, and PEEP of 0.

34. What is the most likely diagnosis? Why?

35. With regard to the oxygenation status, what changes would you recommend?

36. With regard to the volume, what changes would you recommend?

Case 2

A 65-year-old, 143-lb (65-kg) woman was intubated after presenting in the emergency department with pulmonary edema and severe respiratory distress. Now she is in the ICU with a temperature of 97° F, blood pressure of 80/50 mm Hg, heart rate of 120 beats/min, and SpO_2 of 90% on 60% oxygen. Her pulmonary capillary wedge pressure is 24 mm Hg and cardiac output is 3 L/min. Breath sounds reveal coarse crackles throughout the lungs. The patient is intubated and currently being ventilated with a tidal volume of 700 ml, frequency of 14, and PEEP of 10 cm H_2O.

37. What is the most likely diagnosis? What's the underlying cause?

38. With regard to the oxygenation status, what changes would you recommend?

WHAT DOES THE NBRC SAY?

Circle the best answer.

39. Which of the following would be useful in treating an elevated shunt in a patient with ARDS who is being mechanically ventilated?
    A. Initiating IMV mode
    B. Optimizing PEEP
    C. Increasing the F_1O_2
    D. Adding expiratory retard

40. Which of the following indicates the optimal PEEP setting?

	PEEP	PaO$_2$	Cardiac Output
A.	5 cm H$_2$O	53 mm Hg	4.5 L/min
B.	10 cm H$_2$O	60 mm Hg	4.3 L/min
C.	15 cm H$_2$O	74 mm Hg	3.8 L/min
D.	20 cm H$_2$O	88 mm Hg	3.4 L/min

41. A patient is admitted to the ICU with a diagnosis of pulmonary edema. Which of the following breath sounds is consistent with this diagnosis?
    A. Inspiratory stridor
    B. Inspiratory crackles
    C. Expiratory rhonchi
    D. Pleural friction rub

42. A patient with ARDS is being ventilated with the following settings:

Mode	Assist Control
F$_1$O$_2$	0.80
Frequency	10
PEEP	5 cm H$_2$O
V$_T$	500 ml
SpO$_2$	82%

Whichof the following would you recommend as possible ways to improve oxygenation?
    A. Increase the tidal volume.
    B. Increase the PEEP.
    C. Increase the F$_1$O$_2$.
    D. Increase the rate.

43. Which of the following would provide necessary information regarding fluid management in a critically ill patient with cardiogenic pulmonary edema?
    A. Bedside pulmonary function testing
    B. Intake and output measurements
    C. Daily weights
    D. Pulmonary artery catheter

44. Chest radiograph changes associated with noncardiogenic pulmonary edema include _____.
    1. pleural effusion
    2. bilateral infiltrates
    3. enlarged left ventricle
       A. 1 and 2 only
       B. 2 only
       C. 2 and 3 only
       D. 1 and 3 only

FOOD FOR THOUGHT

45. Lower inflection point (LIP or P$_{flex}$) is useful in setting appropriate PEEP and tidal volume levels. What is meant by the term LIP? How is it determined?

30 Trauma, Burns and Near Drowning

Match the correct definition with the correct term.

Terms	Definitions
1. _____ Penetrating trauma	A. Laryngospasm with closure of the glottis prevents aspiration of large amounts of fluid in the lungs.
2. _____ Blunt trauma	B. Occur(s) with sudden immersion in water cooler than 25° C.
3. _____ Morbid obesity	C. Scale used to assess traumatic brain injury.
4. _____ Obesity hypoventilation syndrome	D. Multifocal fractures of one or more ribs.
5. _____ Dry drowning	E. BMI greater than 45 kg/m².
6. _____ Wet drowning	F. High force applied to a small surface area of the body, such as with a gunshot.
7. _____ Glasgow Coma Scale	G. Occurs when laryngospasm lessens with unconsciousness, leading to the aspiration of fluid.
8. _____ Tension pneumothorax	H. Affects the most severely obese patients who acquire a reduced chemosensitivity, impairing their ventilatory response to hypoxemia and hypercapnia.
9. _____ Flail chest	I. Develops when the pleural lesion acts as a one-way valve allowing the entrance of air into the pleural space and progressively trapping air in the expanding pleural cavity.
10. _____ Cold shock cardiac-respiratory reflexes	J. High force applied over a larger body surface, such as in the case of a head-on motor vehicle accident.

LIFE-THREATENING TRAUMA

11. How many yearly hospital admissions in the United States are the result of trauma?

12. What are the three categories of the Glasgow Coma Scale?

A. _____

B. _____

C. _____

HEAD, NECK, AND UPPER AIRWAY INJURIES

13. If blunt force trauma is suspected, what intervention should the RT and the medical team perform immediately?

14. You are the RT working in the emergency department of a Level-1 trauma center when a patient presents with blunt trauma to the thoracic region. What are you worried about?

15. What therapeutic approach would you take to manage the patient in Question #14?

OBESITY

16. Fill in the chart below categorizing the Body Mass Index of an individual.

BMI category	Range
Normal BMI	
Obesity	
Severe obesity	
Morbid obesity	
Super obesity	

17. List four diseases associated with obesity.

A. _____

B. _____

C. _____

D. _____

18. What is one of the most challenging aspects of ventilatory management of obese patients?

NEAR DROWNING

19. How many drowning deaths occurred in the United States between 2005 and 2009. In adults, what was the general cause? How many drowning deaths occurred in children under the age of 14?

20. Explain the cold shock cardiac reflexes.

21. What effects does the inhalation of fresh water have on the respiratory system?

22. What effects does the inhalation of salt water have on the respiratory system?

BURNS

23. What three categories does the respiratory assessment of a burn patient include?

    A. _____

    B. _____

    C. _____

24. How effective is a pulse oximeter in measuring arterial oxygen saturation in an inhalation injury?

CASE STUDY

Bastian is a 26-year-old male patient who was involved in a motor vehicle crash. He was not wearing a seat belt and sustained significant chest trauma as well as a broken tibia. He has been stabilized and is in the intensive care unit. He is currently unable to get out of bed.

25. What respiratory complications is Bastian at risk of developing?

26. Bastian's nurse reports to you that he is having trouble clearing his secretions. What is a likely cause for his difficulty?

27. During rounds the next day the attending physician asks for your respiratory treatment plan for Bastian. What interventions would you discuss with the attending physician?

SUMMARY CHECKLIST

28. Any clinical signs of upper airway injury from smoke inhalation generally require _____ and mechanical ventilation.

29. All obese patients should be assessed for sleep apnea and _____ _____ _____.

30. Generally, gas exchange abnormalities in near drowning are a result of fluid shifts and the activation of

_____ _____.

WHAT DOES THE NBRC SAY?

31. Your patient was just intubated following a house fire that resulted in an inhalation injury. What should you set the FiO_2 at when the patient is placed on mechanical ventilation?
    A. 0.5
    B. 0.6
    C. 0.8
    D. 1.0

32. A patient was intubated and mechanically ventilated following a stab wound to the chest. Suddenly, the high-pressure alarm is triggered and simultaneously the patient's heart rate increases and blood pressure drops. What is the likely cause?
    A. Inappropriately set alarms on the ventilator.
    B. A hemopneumothorax has developed.
    C. Acute bronchospasm.
    D. Pleural effusion.

33. Most adult drownings are a result of
    A. diving injury.
    B. alcohol.
    C. inability to swim.
    D. swift water currents.

FOOD FOR THOUGHT

34. Why is early tracheostomy often advocated in burn patients with suspected inhalation injuries?

31 Lung Cancer

WORD WIZARD

Match each of the following abbreviations with its definition.

1.	MRI	A. Staging system based on the size of the tumor, the presence and position of abnormal lymph nodes, and the presence or absence of metastasis.
2.	CT	B. Radiographic techniques that produce a film that represents a detailed cross-section of tissue structure.
3.	TNM	C. Imaging technique using magnetic disturbance of tissue to obtain images.
4.	PET	D. Computerized radiographic technique that uses radioactive substances to examine the metabolic activity of various body structures.

MEET THE OBJECTIVES

5. How many cases of bronchogenic carcinoma were newly diagnosed in the United States in 2014? How many cases does the WHO estimate occur worldwide each year?

   A. _____

   B. _____

6. What percentage of cancer deaths are caused by smoking tobacco?

7. Compare lung cancer deaths of men and women in the United States.

8. What percentage of the total population in the United States smokes? Which group of smokers is the largest? (Which group are you in?)

   A. Percent of population: Men _____ Women _____

   B. Most smokers: _____

   C. Are we winning the war against tobacco?

9. What is another name for passive exposure to smoke?

10. Describe the health risks of passive exposure to smoke.

11. Besides smoking, list four other major influences linked to an increase in lung cancer.

   A. _____

   B. _____

   C. _____

   D. _____

12. What is meant by the term *"apoptosis"*?

13. List the four major histopathologic types of lung cancer along with the epidemiology they represent and a brief description of the cells.

TYPE OF CANCER	EPIDEMIOLOGY	DESCRIPTION
A. Adenocarcinoma		
B. Squamous cell		
C. Large cell		
D. Small cell		

CLINICAL FEATURES

14. List the four common sites of metastasis of cancer originating in the lungs.

   A. _____

   B. _____

   C. _____

   D. _____

15. What percentage of patients with lung cancer is asymptomatic at time of presentation?

16. Local tumor growth in the central airways may cause many symptoms. Name four that a respiratory therapist could easily recognize.

   A. _____

   B. _____

   C. _____

   D. _____

17. Patients with pleural or chest wall involvement will typically have what two symptoms?

A. _____

B. _____

18. Explain "Pancoast syndrome."

19. Give three examples of paraneoplastic syndromes commonly associated with lung cancers. Describe briefly, please.

A.

B.

C.

DIAGNOSIS

20. Two methods are used to obtain tissue for confirmation. Please describe both of the following.
A. Flexible bronchoscopy (FB):

B. Transthoracic needle biopsy (TNB):

21. Why is tumor staging so important?

22. How is small cell cancer staged?

23. What's the consensus on mass screenings for people at high risk for lung cancer?

TREATMENT

24. Why is surgical resection the treatment of choice for all non–small-cell lung cancers?

25. What patients are *not* candidates for surgery in terms of staging?

26. How are respiratory therapists involved in determining candidates for surgery?

27. What test values for percent predicted postoperative (PPO) and D_{LCO} suggest a patient may (or may not!) safely undergo lobectomy or pneumonectomy?

28. Name the two nonsurgical therapy modalities.

A. _____

B. _____

29. What is meant by *palliative* therapy? Give examples.
    A. Medications:

    B. Radiotherapy:

    C. Bronchoscopy:

ROLE OF THE RESPIRATORY THERAPIST

Respiratory therapists don't perform surgery or administer chemotherapy or radiation to cancer patients. Still, many of these patients have preexisting lung disease or have airway problems.

30. Describe the role RTs play in the following.
    A. Nicotine intervention:

    B. Diagnosis:

    C. Support:

Complete the following sentences by writing the correct term(s) in the spaces provided.

31. _____ carcinoma is the leading cause of cancer deaths in the United States.

32. The _____ classification groups patients in stages or categories that correlate

    with _____.

33. The most effective way to prevent lung cancer is to prevent

CASE STUDIES

Chapter 31 has excellent case studies in the form of Mini-Clinis. Four of these cases
are particularly useful to the respiratory therapist.

Pancoast's Tumor 31-1

34. Will you be caring for patients with weakness and drooping eyelids? How is care
    different?

Paraneoplastic Syndrome 31-3

35. Confusion and generalized weakness are signs of what type of serious neurologic
    vascular accident?

Evaluating Surgical Risk 31-5

36. What therapy modalities might improve lung function prior to surgery for lung
    resection?

37. What methods of diagnosis might be useful for the patient with copious amounts of clear, frothy sputum?

FOOD FOR THOUGHT

38. Besides lung cancer, what are the other significant health risks of smoking?

39. With the high incidence and known risk factors for lung cancer, you would expect to see screening techniques available. Discuss this issue.

40. What is brachytherapy?

32 Neuromuscular and Other Diseases of the Chest Wall

Try matching these diseases to their definitions.

Diseases	Definitions
1. _____ Ankylosing spondylitis	A. Neuromuscular conduction disorder that particularly affects the face, throat, and respiratory muscles.
2. _____ Amyotrophic lateral sclerosis	B. Chronic inflammatory disease that fuses the spine and affected joints.
3. _____ Flail chest	C. Muscle wasting disease characterized by delayed relaxation of contracted groups.
4. _____ Guillain-Barré syndrome	D. Degenerative disease of motor neurons characterized by progressive atrophy.
5. _____ Lambert-Eaton syndrome	E. Inflammation of muscles caused by a rheumatologic disorder.
6. _____ Myasthenia gravis	F. Unstable chest as a result of rib fractures that exhibits paradoxical movement on inspiration.
7. _____ Myotonic dystrophy	G. Idiopathic polyneuritis characterized by ascending weakness.
8. _____ Polymyositis	H. Abnormal curvature of the spine that may compromise ventilation.
9. _____ Kyphoscoliosis	I. Neuromuscular conduction disorder associated with underlying malignancy.

MEET THE OBJECTIVES

10. Neuromuscular abnormalities affect four major groups of muscles that may result in respiratory problems. List these four groups.

    A. _____

    B. _____

    C. _____

    D. _____

11. List the three common complaints of patients with respiratory muscle weakness as a result of neuromuscular disease.

    A. _____

    B. _____

    C. _____

12. Pulmonary function testing of patients with neuromuscular disease and otherwise normal lung tissue will demonstrate what type of ventilatory defect?

13. What three specific tests are most useful in monitoring ventilatory function in patients with neuromuscular weakness?

   A. Assess volumes with _____

   B. Assess muscle strength via _____

   C. Assess hypoxemia and hypercapnia with _____

14. What signs and symptoms suggest performing nocturnal oximetry or formal sleep testing?

15. What is the primary treatment for severe respiratory muscle weakness? What is diaphragmatic pacing?

   A. Primary treatment: _____

   B. Diaphragmatic pacing: _____

SPECIFIC NEUROMUSCULAR DISEASES

16. What is myopathic disease? Give two examples of common myopathies.

   A. What is it? _____

   B. Example 1 _____

   C. Example 2 _____

17. What general category of drugs is used to treat myasthenia gravis?

18. What surgical treatment may be effective in some cases of myasthenia gravis?

19. List four predisposing factors to Guillain-Barré syndrome (GBS).

   A. _____

   B. _____

   C. _____

   D. _____

20. Bilateral interruption of the phrenic nerves that results in diaphragmatic paralysis is seen in what type of injury?

21. Reversible unilateral diaphragmatic paralysis occurs frequently following what commonly performed surgery?

22. Describe the chest radiographic presentation of unilateral diaphragmatic paralysis.

23. Define the high and middle/low classification of cervical cord lesions.

    A. High: _____

    B. Middle/low: _____

24. Describe the muscle groups affected by each of the following spine injuries.

	Level	Muscle Groups
A.	C1-2	_____
B.	C3-5	_____
C.	C4-8	_____
D.	T1-12	_____
E.	T7-L1	_____

25. What type of breathing is the hallmark sign of significant diaphragmatic weakness?

26. What are the two basic types of strokes?

    A. _____

    B. _____

27. Give examples of the effect on the respiratory system of strokes in the following locations in the brain.

Location	Effect on Respiration
A. Cerebral cortex	_____
B. Bilateral hemispheric infarct	_____
C. Lateral medulla	_____
D. Mid pons	_____

28. Aside from problems similar to stroke, brain trauma can cause what respiratory "fluid" problems?

    A. _____

    B. _____

29. Describe these two chest wall deformations that often occur together.
    A. Kyphosis:

    B. Scoliosis:

30. Describe the ventilatory defects and pulmonary function changes associated with severe kyphoscoliosis.
    A. Ventilation:

    B. Pulmonary function:

31. Describe the paradoxical chest motion that is the hallmark of flail chest.

32. Name three other pulmonary injuries frequently associated with flail chest.

    A. _____

    B. _____

    C. _____

33. Regardless of the physiologic mechanisms behind respiratory dysfunction, what are the mainstays of treatment for flail chest?

A. _____

B. _____

C. _____

SUMMARY CHECKLIST

Complete the following sentences by writing the correct term(s) in the spaces provided.

34. Weakness and _____ failure are the most important respiratory dysfunctions in many neuromuscular diseases.

35. Signs and symptoms of muscle weakness include exertional _____ orthopnea, soft vocalizations, and a

weak _____.

36. PFTs typically show a decreased _____ lung capacity, decreased _____ capacity, and

decreased _____ inspiratory pressures.

CASE STUDIES

Case 1

A 27-year-old woman was admitted from her physician's office following complaints of fatigue. Upon interview, the patient reports that she becomes weak after any exertion, especially in her arms. She also complains of difficulty swallowing. She denies any recent illness. Vital signs show a normal temperature and slightly increased heart rate and respiration. Inspection reveals that she has drooping eyelids and appears to have little tone in her facial muscles.

37. Based on this information, what is the most likely diagnosis?

38. What drug therapy might help to confirm this diagnosis?

39. Why is measurement of inspiratory and expiratory pressures a more sensitive test of muscle function than measurement of vital capacity?

A 52-year-old man was admitted from his physician's office following complaints of fatigue. Upon interview, he reports that his feet felt numb yesterday and that his legs were weak when he got up this morning. He went to the physician because he thought he might be having a stroke. He states that he had the flu about 2 weeks earlier. Vital signs show a normal temperature and slightly increased heart rate and respiration.

40. Based on this information, what neuromuscular condition is likely?

41. How would analysis of CSF be useful in making a diagnosis?

42. What two treatment strategies have improved outcome in this syndrome?

A. _____

B. _____

WHAT DOES THE NBRC SAY?

Circle the best answer.

43. A 23-year-old patient with flail chest is transferred to the ICU for observation following a motor vehicle accident. After 2 hours, the patient complains of increasing dyspnea, and arterial blood gas analysis is performed.

pH   7.27
$PaCO_2$ 55 mm Hg
PaO_2 61 mm Hg

What action should the respiratory therapist recommend at this time?
A. Place the patient on oxygen therapy.
B. Initiate mask CPAP.
C. Administer a bronchodilator drug.
D. Initiate mechanical ventilation.

44. A patient with Guillain-Barré syndrome has had serial vital capacity measurements.

0900   3.1 L
1100   2.6 L
1300   2.1 L
1500   1.6 L

In regard to these data, what should the respiratory therapist recommend?
A. Increase the monitoring to every hour.
B. Administer Tensilon.
C. Provide intubation and mechanical ventilation.
D. Continue to monitor the patient every 2 hours.

45. A vital capacity below what value indicates the need for intubation and ventilation in a patient with acute neuromuscular disease?
    A. 30 ml/kg
    B. 20 ml/kg
    C. 15 ml/kg
    D. 10 ml/kg

46. A patient with myasthenia gravis presents in the emergency department with profound muscle weakness. Administration of which of the following will improve ventilation?
    A. Pancuronium
    B. Neostigmine
    C. Epinephrine
    D. Atropine

47. The presence of paradoxical chest motion on inspiration following a motor vehicle accident most likely indicates

    _____
    A. flail chest
    B. pulmonary contusion
    C. pneumothorax
    D. hypoxemia

FOOD FOR THOUGHT

48. ALS is a disease that strikes down heroes in the prime of life. Prognosis is poor. A newly approved therapy for ALS is riluzole. Please discuss.
    A. Riluzole:

33 Disorders of Sleep

Give the full name for each of the following acronyms from Chapter 33.

1. BiPAP: _____
2. CSA: _____
3. CPAP: _____
4. RDI: _____
5. EEG: _____
6. EPAP: _____
7. IPAP: _____
8. OSA: _____
9. PSG: _____
10. UPPP: _____
11. AHI: _____

MEET THE OBJECTIVES

12. What is the definition of sleep apnea? What about hypopnea?

13. Explain how OSA differs from CSA.

14. What is the estimated incidence of OSA in the adult population?

15. Why does airway closure occur during sleep?

16. List five adverse cardiopulmonary consequences of untreated OSA.

    A. _____

    B. _____

    C. _____

    D. _____

    E. _____

17. List two neurobehavioral and two metabolic consequences of untreated OSA.
    Neurobehavioral

    A. _____

    B. _____

    Metabolic

    C. _____

    D. _____

18. List three factors that predispose a patient to OSA.

    A. _____

    B. _____

    C. _____

19. Describe the six common clinical features seen in many cases of OSA.

    A. _____

    B. _____

    C. _____

    D. _____

    E. _____

    F. _____

20. What is the current gold standard for making a diagnosis of OSA?

21. What value of the apnea-hypopnea index is consistent with moderate to severe sleep apnea? What is considered normal?

22. What are the three goals of treatment for OSA?

A. _____

B. _____

C. _____

23. Discuss the behavioral options that should be pursued in all patients with sleep-disordered breathing.

24. Why do you think nocturnal CPAP has become the first-line medical therapy for OSA?

25. How does CPAP work to relieve OSA?

26. What is auto-titrating CPAP?

27. Identify the indications and explain how the titration of bilevel positive airway pressure therapy differs from that of CPAP.

28. Describe five of the common minor side effects of positive-pressure therapy. Identify what you can do to help the patient solve these annoying problems.

   A. _____

   B. _____

   C. _____

   D. _____

   E. _____

29. What is the role of tracheostomy in treating sleep apnea?

30. What is the success rate of UPPP, and what is the current recommendation regarding this procedure as a treatment for OSA?

SUMMARY CHECKLIST

Identify the key points from Chapter 33. Complete the following questions by writing the correct term(s) in the spaces provided.

31. The three types of sleep apnea are obstructive, _____, and _____.

32. The predominant risk factor for airway narrowing or closure during sleep is a _____ or

    _____ upper airway.

33. The long-term adverse consequences of OSA include poor _____ functioning as well as increased risk

    of _____ morbidity and mortality.

34. Risk factors for OSA include _____ gender, age greater than _____ years, upper body _____, and habitual _____.

35. The first-line medical therapy for OSA is _____.

36. _____ positive airway pressure therapy may be useful in salvaging patients who have difficulty complying with CPAP.

37. _____ therapy may be an option for a select group of patients who have undergone extensive upper airway analysis and do comply with medical therapy.

WHAT DOES THE NBRC SAY?

Circle the best answer.

38. An RT notes in the medical record that a patient is receiving BiPAP therapy with a machine he brought from home. Which of the following is the most likely diagnosis for the patient?
    A. Pulmonary emphysema
    B. Congestive heart failure
    C. Obstructive sleep apnea
    D. Central sleep apnea

39. A sleep study shows simultaneous cessation of airflow and respiratory muscle effort. These findings are consistent with _____
    A. pulmonary hypertension
    B. obstructive sleep apnea
    C. congestive heart failure
    D. central sleep apnea

40. Which of the following is *true* regarding BiPAP therapy?
    1. Expiratory pressure is always set above inspiratory pressure.
    2. BiPAP units are pneumatically powered.
    3. BiPAP should be increased until snoring ceases.
       A. 1 and 3 only
       B. 2 only
       C. 2 and 3 only
       D. 3 only

FOOD FOR THOUGHT

If you want to gain more professional expertise on this subject, look no further than the journal *Respiratory Care*, which has editions devoted only to sleep-disordered breathing!

34 Neonatal and Pediatric Respiratory Disorders

WORD WIZARD

Try this matching exercise to test your ability to understand the new terms and acronyms found in Chapter 34.

Terms	Definitions
1. _____ RDS	A. Poor clearance of lung fluids
2. _____ Croup	B. Aspiration of fetal feces
3. _____ GERD	C. Chronic problem from alveolar trauma and oxygen toxicity
4. _____ PPHN	D. Life-threatening upper airway infection
5. _____ MAS	E. Virus-induced subglottic swelling
6. _____ TTN	F. Acute infection of the lower airways
7. _____ SIDS	G. Leading cause of death in infants < 1 year old
8. _____ Epiglottitis	H. Complex syndrome of newborn hypertension
9. _____ BPD	I. Stomach problem associated with asthma
10. _____ Bronchiolitis	J. Surfactant deficiency in preemies

BABY BLUES

11. How many babies in the United States have RDS?

12. What is the primary pathophysiology in infants with RDS?

13. Describe the four clinical signs of RDS that are listed below.

   A. Respiratory rate: _____

   B. Breathing pattern: _____

   C. Auscultation: _____

   D. Audible sounds: _____

14. How is a definitive diagnosis for RDS usually made?

15. Discuss the four main therapies for treating RDS.
    A. CPAP: Starting values? Device?

    B. Ventilator: When do you start? What is the goal of PEEP for this baby?

    C. Surfactant: When to give? Positioning?

    D. HFV: What does this acronym mean?

16. How does the chest radiograph of a baby with transient tachypnea of the newborn (TTN) (type II RDS) differ from that of primary RDS?

17. List two typical respiratory treatments for TTN.

    A. _____

    B. _____

18. Meconium aspiration is usually associated with what fetal event?

19. MAS usually occurs in infants of what age?

20. Name the three primary problems in MAS.

    A. _____

    B. _____

    C. _____

21. Immediate treatment of the MAS baby is vital! What should you do?

    A. Upon delivery: _____

    B. Repeat until: _____

    C. If the condition worsens: _____

22. In some ways, bronchopulmonary dysplasia is a result of our efforts to save preterm infants. What are the five events implicated in causing BPD?

    A. _____

    B. _____

    C. _____

    D. _____

    E. _____

23. What is the "best management" of BPD, and how and where does this begin?

    A. Best: _____

    B. How: _____

    C. Where: _____

24. Please define "periodic breathing," and compare that to "abnormal apneic spells."
    A. Periodic breathing:

    B. Abnormal apneic spells:

25. Describe how the following strategies work to alleviate infant apneic events.
    A. Tactile stimulation:

    B. CPAP:

    C. Caffeine (xanthines):

    D. Doxapram (Dopram):

    E. Transfusion:

26. Describe the basic idea behind each of these treatments for PPHN.
    A. Oxygen

    B. Glucose

    C. Inotropes

    D. Sedation

    E. HFV

    F. Inhaled NO

    G. ECMO

27. List the four defects seen in tetralogy of Fallot.

    A. _____

    B. _____

    C. _____

    D. _____

28. Acyanotic heart diseases are also seen in newborns. PDA is of special interest to RTs. Describe PDA. Name two treatments.

A. Description:

B. Treatments:

C. Explain the use of two pulse oximeters in this situation. You'll need to look back at PPHN to find the answer.

PEDIATRIC PROBLEMS

29. Describe the typical profile of a baby who dies of SIDS.

30. What sleeping position is strongly linked with SIDS?

31. Identify the six infant characteristics often seen near the time of death.

A. _____

B. _____

C. _____

D. _____

E. _____

F. _____

32. What is gastroesophageal reflux disease (GERD)? Name a few of the many respiratory problems this condition can trigger.

33. What age group of kids typically develops bronchiolitis?

34. RSV is one particularly nasty virus that's the culprit in many cases of bronchiolitis. Discuss:
   A. Immunization. Who gets it?

   _____

   B. What does RSV stand for?

   _____

   C. How is the diagnosis made?

   _____

35. Dyspnea, tachypnea, wheezing, and cough are common in these kids. If they have to be hospitalized, what respiratory treatments are indicated?

   A. Bronchodilators, recommended or not recommended? _____

   B. Why give antibiotics for a virus? _____

   C. Hygiene? _____

CASE STUDIES

Case 1

A mother brings her previously healthy 1-year-old to the ED. She states that her baby had a cold 2 days ago, but he still has a slight fever and has been coughing. Mom became concerned when she heard audible wheezing. A treatment with albuterol in the ED has had no effect. Vital signs are essentially normal, except for a slight elevation in respiratory rate. The chest radiograph shows mild hyperinflation with no signs of consolidation. Pulse oximetry shows a saturation of 94%.

36. What diagnosis is most likely?

37. How can a diagnosis of RSV be ruled out?

38. The physician decides to send mom and baby home. What treatment would you recommend?

A 3-year-old is brought to the ED with respiratory distress and a barking cough. The child has been sick for several days with a low-grade fever and stuffy nose. Examination reveals moderate inspiratory stridor and retractions. The pulse oximeter shows a saturation of 88% on room air. A lateral neck film identifies subglottic narrowing with a "steeple sign."

39. What is the most likely diagnosis?

40. What aerosolized medication is traditionally delivered?

41. When should you add nebulized budesonide?

42. How would you deliver oxygen to this child?

A 5-year-old is brought to the emergency department with labored breathing and a high fever. Examination reveals marked inspiratory stridor. The child is listless, and dad says he has had a sore throat. When you talk to the boy, he responds very quietly with short answers. A lateral neck radiograph identifies a "thumb sign."

43. What is the most likely diagnosis?

44. What organism is usually responsible for this condition? How could you confirm?

45. What is the immediate treatment for this condition? Who should perform the intervention and where?

46. What should not be done?

A woman brings her 2-year-old grandson into the clinic because "his breathing just isn't right." She states, "This boy is coughing all the time. Besides, he isn't growing very well, and when I kiss him his skin tastes salty!"

47. How would your diagnosis be confirmed? What values indicate CF?

48. What dietary modifications are needed in cystic fibrosis?

49. List four respiratory treatments aimed at decreasing airway obstruction.

   A. _____

   B. _____

   C. _____

   D. _____

50. Nebulizing drugs are one of the key treatments in this situation. Tell me more about:
   A. Mucolytic drugs:

   B. 7% solution:

   C. What are tobramycin and aztreonam?

WHAT DOES THE NBRC SAY?

Circle the best answer.

51. A premature infant is experiencing episodes of apnea and cyanosis. The respiratory therapist should recommend which of the following?
   A. Albuterol
   B. Narcan
   C. Exosurf
   D. Caffeine

52. A 5-year-old child presents in the ED with complaints of a severe sore throat. The child has inspiratory stridor and muffled phonation. He has a fever of 40° C. His mother states he will not drink anything, so she brought him in.

The most likely diagnosis is _____
A. croup
B. bronchiolitis
C. foreign body aspiration
D. epiglottitis

53. Which of the following tests is helpful in establishing a diagnosis of cystic fibrosis?
A. Sweat chloride
B. L/S ratio
C. Apgar score
D. Pneumogram

54. Which of the following is the most appropriate imaging technique to help confirm a diagnosis of croup?
A. Computed tomogram
B. PA chest film
C. Lateral neck film
D. Bronchogram

55. A 4-year-old child with LTB presents in the ED with moderate stridor and harsh breath sounds. The RT should recommend which of the following?
A. Albuterol
B. Racemic epinephrine
C. Immediate intubation
D. Aminophylline

FOOD FOR THOUGHT

Many students ask, "What's the difference between an infant, baby, child . . .?" Here are some definitions for you that are not in *Egan's*:
- **Fetus:** The unborn offspring from the end of the eighth week after conception (when the major structures have formed) until birth. Up until the eighth week, the developing offspring is called an embryo.
- **Premature baby:** A baby born before 37 weeks of gestation have passed. Historically, the definition of prematurity was 2500 grams (about 5½ pounds) or less at birth. The current World Health Organization definition of prematurity is a baby born before 37 weeks of gestation.
- **Neonate:** This is a newborn baby. If the baby leaves the newborn nursery, goes home, and comes back to the hospital, he or she may be put into the pediatric unit.
- **Postterm baby:** A postterm baby is born 2 weeks (14 days) or more after the usual 9 months (280 days) of gestation.
- **Child:** This is a person 6 to 12 years of age. An individual 2 to 5 years old is a preschool-aged child. Sometimes we use the following criteria: Ages 1 to 8 for a child. Obviously size is important when you're talking about ET tubes and drug dosages, because some children are quite large. When a child is the physical size of an adult, you would use adult dosages.

Chapter **34** **Neonatal and Pediatric Respiratory Disorders**

35 Airway Pharmacology

WORD WIZARD

Try this matching exercise to test your ability to understand the new terms found in Chapter 35. (You may have to really dig for some of these—use the chapter, the glossary, and a medical dictionary if necessary!)

Terms	Definitions
1. _____ Indication	A. Time it takes to metabolize half of a drug dose.
2. _____ Tolerance	B. Drug may not be given for any reason.
3. _____ Adrenergic	C. Effect of acetylcholine on smooth muscle.
4. _____ Vasopressor	D. Reason for giving a drug to a patient.
5. _____ Prodrug	E. Undesired effect of a drug.
6. _____ Muscarinic	F. Drugs that mimic the effect of epinephrine.
7. _____ Pharmacodynamic	G. Has receptor affinity and exerts an effect.
8. _____ Side effect	H. Mimics the effect of acetylcholine.
9. _____ Absolute contraindication	I. Drug that exerts a constricting effect on blood vessels.
10. _____ Leukotriene	J. Given in an inactive form that converts to active in the body.
11. _____ Mydriasis	K. Dilation of the pupil of the eye.
12. _____ Agonist	L. Phase related to mechanism of action.
13. _____ Pharmacokinetic	M. Maximum effect from a drug dose.
14. _____ Cholinergic	N. Time it takes a drug to start working.
15. _____ Antagonist	O. How long a drug's effect lasts.
16. _____ Tachyphylaxis	P. Increasing dose needed for effect.
17. _____ Onset	Q. Has receptor affinity but produces no effect.
18. _____ Peak effect	R. Rapidly developing tolerance.
19. _____ Duration	S. Compounds that produce allergic or inflammatory responses.
20. _____ Half-life	T. Phase related to metabolism of a drug.

JUST SAY YES

21. What is the most common medication route of administration that is used by RTs?

22. List four advantages of this route.

A. _____

B. _____

C. _____

D. _____

23. List two disadvantages of this route.

A. _____

B. _____

24. How do medications delivered by this route usually end up in the systemic circulation?

25. Describe the two primary divisions of the autonomic nervous system in terms of name, main neurotransmitter, and effect on bronchial smooth muscle.

	DIVISION	OTHER NAME	NEUROTRANSMITTER	AIRWAY MUSCLE EFFECT
A.	Sympathetic			
B.	Parasympathetic			

ADRENERGIC BRONCHODILATORS

26. State the three receptors of the sympathetic nervous system and their basic effects.

	RECEPTOR	PRIMARY EFFECT
A.		
B.		
C.		

27. Give the generic name, brand name, strength, and dose for the following commonly used beta-adrenergic bronchodilators.

	GENERIC NAME	BRAND NAME	STRENGTH	DOSE
A.	Albuterol SVN			
	Albuterol MDI			
B.	Levalbuterol SVN			
	Levalbuterol MDI			
C.	Salmeterol DPI			
D.	Formoterol DPI			
E.	Arformoterol SVN			
F.	Indacaterol DPI			
G.	Olodaterol DPI			

28. It is especially important that you know how long it takes for a drug to start working and reach its maximum effect and how long the drug will last. Fill in the information for the drugs listed below.

	DRUG	ONSET	PEAK EFFECT	DURATION
A.	Xopenex			
B.	Racemic epinephrine			
C.	Proventil			
D.	Serevent			
E.	Formoterol			
F.	Arformoterol			

29. List the most common side effects of bronchodilator drugs. Which one is the most frequent?

A. _____

B. _____

C. _____

D. _____

30. What vital signs should you monitor when administering any drugs via the aerosol route?

A. _____

B. _____

C. _____

D. _____

E. _____

31. How would you assess long-term bronchodilator use?

A. _____

B. _____

C. _____

D. _____

E. _____

ANTICHOLINERGIC BRONCHODILATORS

32. Generally, ipratropium bromide is indicated for use in patients with what pathology?

33. Fill in the blanks to complete your knowledge of ipratropium bromide and combinations of it with SABA and LABA.

NAME	BRAND NAME	STRENGTH	DOSE
Ipratropium bromide MDI			
Ipratropium bromide SVN			
Ipratropium bromide and albuterol MDI			
Ipratropium bromide and albuterol SVN			
Ipratropium bromide and albuterol SMI			
Tiotropium bromide			

34. Describe the side effects to watch for when administering this class of drugs.
Common side effects

A. _____

B. _____

MDI occasional side effects

A. _____

B. _____

SVN occasional side effects

A. _____

B. _____

MUCUS CONTROLLING AGENTS

35. Describe the mucoactive agents available for nebulization.

	AGENT	BRAND NAME	DOSE	INDICATION
A.	Acetylcysteine 10% or 20%			
B.	Dornase alfa			
C.	Aqueous aerosols			

36. Bronchospasm is a common side effect of the administration of mucolytic agents. How would you recommend modifying the therapy to prevent or treat this problem?

37. What types of short-term and long-term assessments should you make to monitor the effectiveness of these drugs?

INHALED GLUCOCORTICOIDS

38. How long will it take for inhaled steroids to have a noticeable effect on the symptoms of asthma?

39. What significance does this have in terms of patient education?

40. The most common side effects of inhaled steroids are local ones (as opposed to systemic). Name the four most common problems.

A. _____

B. _____

C. _____

D. _____

41. Other than a reservoir device, what two additional recommendations are made by GOLD and NAEPP in regard to corticosteroid inhalers?

42. What would you assess to determine if the steroids were working in the long run?

NONSTEROIDAL ANTIASTHMA DRUGS

43. What is believed to be the mode of action of cromolyn sodium?

44. List the number one side effect for each of the following:

    A. Zafirlukast (Accolate): _____

    B. Zileuton (Zyflo): _____

    C. Montelukast (Singulair): _____

TREATING INFECTION BY THE AEROSOL ROUTE

45. What agent may be nebulized to treat *P. jiroveci* (formerly called PCP or *Pneumocystis carinii* pneumonia) seen in severely immunocompromised patients?

46. What are the common undesired respiratory side effects of administration? What modification of therapy would you recommend if they occur?

47. While *P. jiroveci* (PCP) is not a hazard to healthy people, patients with AIDS often have what other disease that is transmitted via the airborne route?

48. Describe the use of ribavirin in terms of indication, patient population, and special equipment needed for administration.

    A. Indication: _____

    B. Type of patient: _____

    C. Nebulizer: _____

    D. Organism: _____

49. What about TOBI?

    A. Drug: _____

    B. Type of patient: _____

    C. Nebulizer: _____

    D. Organism: _____

50. What about Aztreonam?

    A. Drug: _____

    B. Type of patient: _____

    C. Nebulizer: _____

    D. Organism: _____

INFLUENZA

51. Which inhaled drug can shorten the course of influenza and alleviate symptoms? What is the problem with giving it to asthma and COPD patients?

    A. Drug: _____

    B. Problem: _____

    C. Delivery system: _____

    D. What is the "off-label use"?

INHALED VASODILATORS

52. Specifically, when is nitric oxide used for newborns? When is it contraindicated?

53. What is the most common adverse reaction during weaning from nitric oxide? What type of hemoglobin disorder could be monitored?

54. What is the brand name of iloprost? What is the class of drugs it represents? (Be specific.)

    A. _____

    B. _____

55. What nebulizer is used to deliver the drug?

56. Describe treprostinil.

    A. Indications and goal: _____

    B. Delivery system: _____

    C. Mode of action: _____

Case 1

A patient who has asthma is admitted to the hospital for the second time in 2 months. She has not been able to get relief and is using her albuterol inhaler frequently.

57. In addition to inhaled beta agonists, steroids are commonly administered to *reduce* inflammation associated with asthma. Name one inhaled steroid and recommend a dosage.

58. What device is important to use along with MDIs to prevent deposition of these drugs in the mouth?

59. Why should this patient rinse her mouth after use of her inhaled steroid?

60. What long-acting bronchodilator may help this patient sleep through the night without being awakened by dyspnea and wheezing?

Case 2

Cystic fibrosis is diagnosed in a 7-year-old. This patient has extremely thick mucus (like glue!). Auscultation reveals scattered wheezing and rhonchi.

61. What drug would you recommend aerosolizing for treatment of the thick mucus?

62. What other drug should be given to treat the wheezing?

63. The patient has *Pseudomonas* in his sputum. What could you nebulize to treat gram-negative bad boys in CF?

Case 3

A 67-year-old man with long-standing COPD characterized by chronic bronchitis is coughing up copious amounts of very thick white sputum. He complains that his chest feels tight, and he cannot catch his breath. His albuterol inhaler is not providing relief.

64. What bronchodilator is appropriate to add to the therapeutic regimen?

65. What alternative delivery methods might be useful?

A respiratory care student is administering a standard dose of albuterol via SVN to a 65-year-old male admitted for pneumonia and COPD. Five minutes into the treatment the patient's heart rate increases from 92 to 156 on the monitor. The instructor walks in at this moment.

66. What action should the student do first? What other actions might be taken right away at the bedside?

67. What diagnostic test should be ordered?

68. What change in medication could provide bronchodilation with fewer side effects?

WHAT DOES THE NBRC SAY?

Try these exercises. Circle the best answer.

69. A patient with asthma comes to the emergency department with dyspnea, hypoxemia, and wheezing. The

    appropriate medication at this time is _____.
    A. administration of nitric oxide
    B. nebulized cromolyn sodium
    C. nebulized albuterol (Ventolin)
    D. nebulized ipratropium bromide (Atrovent)

70. Following extubation, a patient has mild stridor. Which of the following would you recommend at this time?
    A. Administration of oxygen
    B. Aerosolized albuterol (Proventil)
    C. Aerosolized virazole (Ribavirin)
    D. Aerosolized racemic epinephrine

71. After administering a corticosteroid via MDI, the RT should ask the patient to perform which of the following actions?
    A. Rinse and gargle with water.
    B. Deep breathe and cough.
    C. Inhale an adrenergic bronchodilator.
    D. Inhale via a spacer device.

72. The heart rate of a patient receiving an adrenergic bronchodilator rises from 80 to 94 beats per minute during the treatment. Which of the following actions is most appropriate?
    A. Discontinue the therapy.
    B. Let the patient rest for 5 minutes.
    C. Continue the treatment.
    D. Reduce the dosage of the bronchodilator.

73. A physician calls in an order for bronchodilator therapy for a patient with COPD. The order states "0.05 ml of

    albuterol in 3 ml of normal saline via SVN four times per day." The RT should _____.
    A. deliver the treatment as ordered
    B. recommend substituting Atrovent
    C. carefully monitor heart rate during the treatment
    D. call the physician to verify the order

74. Which of the following is the most commonly used rescue medication for acute episodes of bronchospasm?
    A. Albuterol
    B. Atrovent
    C. Advair
    D. Primatene

75. A patient's asthma is poorly controlled with bronchodilators and inhaled steroids. This individual has multiple allergies that trigger her asthma. What additional medication could the respiratory therapist recommend to achieve better control?
    A. Methylxanthines
    B. Modifiers
    C. Oral steroids
    D. Nonsteroidal antiinflammatory agents

FOOD FOR THOUGHT

76. Besides treatment of excessively thick mucous, what can Mucomyst be used for?

36 Airway Management

SUCTIONING

1. What is the name of the device commonly used to suction secretions or fluids from the oropharynx?

2. Describe the cause of and how to prevent each of the following complications.

	COMPLICATION	CAUSE	PREVENTION
A.	Hypoxemia		
B.	Cardiac arrhythmia		
C.	Hypotension		
D.	Atelectasis		
E.	Mucosal trauma		
F.	Increased ICP		
G.	Bacterial colonization of lower airway		

3. Discuss the advantages and disadvantages of closed-system multiuse catheters.
   A. Advantages:

   B. Disadvantages:

4. What special catheter is used to facilitate entry into the left mainstem bronchus?

5. What specialized airway is used to facilitate repeated nasal suctioning?

6. What device do you need to include when you want to collect a sputum specimen during suctioning?

7. What type of lung disease requires the use of a double-lumen ET tube?

   _____

   These are also called Carlen's, or endobronchial, tubes. What is the name of the special type of ventilation used with this tube? _____

8. High-frequency jet ventilation tubes look like standard tubes with two additional lines. What are they?

   A. _____

   B. _____

9. Continuous aspiration of subglottic secretions is the generic name for the Hi-Lo Evac Tube. What is the reported benefit of the subglottic suction (i.e., CASS or Hi-Lo Evac) tube?

INTUBATION PROCEDURES

10. What is the preferred route for establishing an emergency tracheal airway?

11. Why is suction equipment needed for intubation?

12. Describe two common troubleshooting procedures used when the laryngoscope does not light up properly.

13. Prior to insertion, how should the RT test the tube?

14. How is the patient's head positioned to align the mouth, pharynx, and larynx?

15. What other actions *must be taken* before making any attempt to intubate?

16. How long should you attempt intubation? Why do you think we have a rule like this one?

17. List at least two anatomic landmarks *in addition to the glottis* that should be visualized prior to intubation.

   A. _____

   B. _____

18. Compare the use of the Miller and Macintosh laryngoscope blades during the intubation procedure.

19. List nine methods for bedside assessment of correct tube position.

A. _____

B. _____

C. _____

D. _____

E. _____

F. _____

G. _____

H. _____

I. _____

20. What is the disadvantage of using capnographic or colorimetric analysis of carbon dioxide to assess intubation in a cardiac arrest victim?

21. What is the final step of confirmation of endotracheal tube placement?

22. Give two examples of clinical situations where nasotracheal intubation might be preferred over oral intubation.

A. _____

B. _____

23. Describe the two techniques used for nasal intubation.

A. _____

B. _____

24. You may need to use medications to facilitate intubation. What drugs would you use to:
   A. Numb the airway and reflexes

   B. Sedate the patient

   C. Paralyze the patient

TRACHEOTOMY

25. What is the primary indication for performing a tracheotomy?

26. Describe the sequence for removing an ET during the tracheotomy procedure. You might want to remember this procedure!

27. Compare the location of placement in percutaneous and traditional surgical tracheotomy.

28. Name at least three advantages of the percutaneous technique compared with traditional surgical tracheotomy.

   A. _____
   B. _____
   C. _____

29. Compare the following laryngeal injuries associated with intubation in terms of symptoms and treatment.

	INJURY	SYMPTOMS	TREATMENT
A.	Glottic edema		
B.	Vocal cord inflammation		
C.	Laryngeal ulceration		
D.	Polyp/granuloma		
E.	Vocal cord paralysis		
F.	Laryngeal stenosis		

30. Describe the tracheoesophageal fistula in terms of cause, complications, and treatment.

31. Tracheoinnominate fistula is a rare but serious complication. What are the clues, and what are the immediate and corrective actions to take?

What is the survival rate?

CARE OF AN ARTIFICIAL AIRWAY

32. What is the most common material used to secure endotracheal tubes? Tracheostomy tubes?

What is the alternative?

33. How do flexion and extension of the neck affect tube motion? What is the average distance the tube will move (in cm)?

34. What is a "talking" trach? What are some of the problems with these devices?

35. When using a Passy-Muir Valve, what do you need to do with the cuff? How about the ventilator?

HUMIDIFICATION

36. What is the worst problem that results from inadequate humidification of the artificial airway?

37. What temperature range must be maintained in a heated humidification system to provide adequate inspired moisture?

38. What device can be used as an alternative to heated humidifiers for short-term humidification of the intubated patient?

39. What is the most common cause of airway obstruction in the critically ill patient?

CUFF CARE

40. What is the recommended safe cuff pressure? What is the consequence of elevated cuff pressures?

41. What may happen when the tube is too small for the patient's trachea?

TRACH CARE

42. Briefly describe the eight basic steps of tracheotomy care.

A. _____

B. _____

C. _____

D. _____

E. _____

F. _____

G. _____

H. _____

AIRWAY EMERGENCIES

43. List three airway emergencies.

    A. _____

    B. _____

    C. _____

44. List four possible reasons why a tube may become obstructed.

    A. _____

    B. _____

    C. _____

    D. _____

45. What simple technique is used to assess tube obstructions that are not relieved by repositioning the head or deflating the cuff?

46. If you cannot clear the obstruction, what action should you be prepared to take?

47. What additional troubleshooting step can often be performed on patients with tracheostomies?

48. What effects will occur with a cuff leak when a patient is being mechanically ventilated?

EXTUBATION AND DECANNULATION

49. The decision to remove the airway and the decision to remove the ventilator are not the same. What kinds of patients might need to remain intubated even after the ventilator is removed?

50. Describe the method for performing a "cuff-leak test."
    What does *Egan's* suggest as a percentage of leak that should lead to considering extubation?

51. List five types of equipment you will want to assemble *prior* to extubation.

    A. _____

    B. _____

    C. _____

    D. _____

    E. _____

251

52. What therapeutic modality is usually applied immediately after extubation?

53. List three of the most common problems that may occur after extubation.

54. A common complication of extubation is glottic edema. How will you recognize *and* treat this problem?

55. List three methods for weaning from a tracheostomy tube. Give one advantage and one disadvantage for each technique. This is national exam material.

	TECHNIQUE	ADVANTAGE	DISADVANTAGE
A.			
B.			
C.			

AIRWAY ALTERNATIVES

56. List three advantages of the LMA.

A. _____

B. _____

C. _____

57. List two disadvantages of the LMA.

A. _____

B. _____

BRONCHOSCOPY

58. List one advantage and three disadvantages of rigid bronchoscope.

59. What drugs would RTs nebulize prior to the procedure on a nonintubated patient? What about after the procedure?

A. Before: _____

B. After: _____

60. What three types of cardiopulmonary monitoring devices are considered essential for this procedure?

A. _____

B. _____

C. _____

61. What are some of the activities RTs might perform while assisting with the procedure?

A. _____

B. _____

C. _____

CASE STUDIES

Case 1

During your first day of clinical training in the ICU, a patient sustains a cardiac arrest. Your clinical instructor asks you to assist in preparing the equipment needed for endotracheal intubation. The patient is a small 56-year-old female.

62. What size endotracheal tube should you select?

63. How should you test the tube prior to insertion?

64. How will you test the laryngoscope and blade for proper function?

65. Once the tube is inserted, how can you quickly assess placement?

Case 2

After your heart-pounding initiation into resuscitation, it is time to check the other ventilator patients in the unit. A 19-year-old woman with a head injury is receiving mechanical ventilation via a cuffed No. 8 tracheostomy tube with an inner cannula. As you enter the room, the high-pressure alarm is sounding.

66. How will you determine the need for suctioning in this situation?

67. What vacuum pressure should be set prior to suctioning?

68. What size suction catheter is suggested using the Rule of Thumb found in *Egan's*?

69. How long, and with what F_IO_2, should you preoxygenate this patient?

Circle the best answer.

70. Which of the following will decrease the risk of damage to the trachea from the endotracheal tube cuff?
    1. Inflating the cuff with less than 10 ml air
    2. Maintaining cuff pressures of 25 cm H_2O
    3. Using a high-volume low-pressure cuff
    4. Inflating the cuff to 25-35 mm Hg
       A. 1 and 2 only
       B. 1 and 3 only
       C. 2 and 3 only
       D. 3 and 4 only

71. The diameter of the suction catheter for an adult should be no larger than
    A. one-tenth the inner diameter of the ET tube.
    B. one-third the inner diameter of the ET tube.
    C. one-half the inner diameter of the ET tube.
    D. three-fourths the inner diameter of the ET tube.

72. A patient with a tracheostomy tube no longer requires mechanical ventilation. Which of the following would facilitate weaning from the tracheostomy tube?
    A. Unfenestrated tracheostomy tube
    B. Cuffed tracheostomy tube
    C. Tracheostomy button
    D. Removal of the inner cannula

73. Extubation is performed on a patient with an endotracheal tube. Presence of which of the following suggests the presence of upper airway edema?
    A. Rhonchi
    B. Crackles
    C. Wheezes
    D. Stridor

74. Which of the following tools is not needed during nasotracheal intubation?
    A. Laryngoscope handle
    B. Stylette
    C. Miller blade
    D. Magill forceps

75. While performing endotracheal suctioning, an RT notes that flow-through is minimal and secretion clearance is sluggish. Which of the following are possible causes of this problem?
    1. The vacuum setting is greater than 120 mm Hg.
    2. The suction canister is full of secretions.
    3. There is a leak in the system.
    4. The tube cuff is overinflated.
       A. 1 and 2 only
       B. 1 and 4 only
       C. 2 and 3 only
       D. 3 and 4 only

76. Rapid, initial determination of endotracheal tube placement can be achieved by _____.
    1. auscultation
    2. arterial blood gas analysis
    3. measurement of end-tidal CO_2
    4. measurement of SpO_2
        A. 1 and 2 only
        B. 1 and 3 only
        C. 2 and 4 only
        D. 3 and 4 only

77. A patient with a tracheostomy tube shows signs of severe airway obstruction. A suction catheter will pass only a short distance into the tube. The RT should _____.
    A. remove the tracheostomy tube
    B. inflate the cuff of the tube
    C. ventilate the tube with positive pressure
    D. remove the inner cannula

78. Which of the following can be used to assess pulmonary circulation during closed-chest cardiac compressions?
    A. Capnometry
    B. Arterial blood gas analysis
    C. Pulse oximetry
    D. Blood pressure monitoring

79. Prior to performing bronchoscopy, an RT is asked to administer a nebulized anesthetic to the patient. What medication is most appropriate to place in the nebulizer?
    A. Versed
    B. Atropine
    C. Morphine
    D. Lidocaine

FOOD FOR THOUGHT

80. Following emergency cricothyroidotomy, when should a definitive airway be established?

37 Emergency Cardiovascular Life Support

WORD WIZARD

Write out the full definition of each acronym below.

1. CABD: _____

2. ACLS: _____

3. AED: _____

4. AHA: _____

5. ARC: _____

6. BLS: _____

7. SCA: _____

8. CDC: _____

9. CNS: _____

10. CPR: _____

11. FBAO: _____

12. EMS: _____

13. NRP: _____

14. PALS: _____

CAUSES AND PREVENTION OF SUDDEN DEATH

15. What is the primary cause of sudden death among adults over the age of 40 in the United States?

16. What is the most common rhythm immediately after cardiac arrest? Briefly describe the two basic treatments.

    A. Rhythm: _____

    B. Treatments: _____

    _____

17. Compare adult, child, and infant resuscitation for the following categories for two rescuers.

	CATEGORY	ADULT	CHILD	INFANT
A.	Compression 1. Hand placement 2. Depth 3. Rate 4. Check pulse			
B.	Obstructed airway 1. Mild 2. Unresponsive			
C.	Ventilation 1. Rate 2. Ratio			

18. You wouldn't want to do CPR on someone who is just sedated. Once you carefully assess unresponsiveness, you need HELP! What should you do in each of these situations?

A. Collapsed outside hospital:

_____

B. In the hospital:

_____

C. How do you quickly check for "signs of life"?

_____

_____

19. When is the jaw-thrust maneuver indicated?

20. How is assessment of pulselessness different in adults and infants?

21. Once CPR is begun, it is normally only stopped for what three reasons?

A. _____

B. _____

C. _____

WHO PUT THE "D" IN DEFIBRILLATION?

22. What is the most likely rhythm of a person with sudden cardiac arrest?

23. Why is early defibrillation so important?

24. Describe the AED briefly. Is the shock really automatic? After hooking up the electrodes, what else is the operator supposed to do?

YES, BUT IS IT GOOD CPR?

25. How can you easily and quickly determine the effectiveness of ventilations and compressions delivered during CPR?

    A. Ventilation: _____

    B. Compression: _____

26. CPR can have complications. State a way to avoid these classics.

    A. Neck injury: _____

    B. Gastric inflation: _____

    C. Vomiting: _____

    D. Internal trauma (liver laceration): _____

    E. FBAO removal: _____

27. CPR is contraindicated under what two circumstances?

    A. _____

    B. _____

28. What barriers does the CDC suggest to protect us during CPR?

FOREIGN BODIES

29. What is the universal distress signal for foreign body obstruction of the airway?

30. Give another name for the abdominal thrust maneuver.

When should you avoid this maneuver in an adult?

What should you do if you cannot or should not perform the abdominal thrust on a choking victim?

31. Describe four ways you can use to determine if the foreign body has been removed from the airway.

A. _____

B. _____

C. _____

D. _____

ADVANCED CARDIAC LIFE SUPPORT

32. What concentration of oxygen should be administered during a life-threatening emergency?

33. What is the technique to select the best-sized oropharyngeal airway (OPA)?

34. What airway would you choose for the patient who cannot tolerate an oral airway?

35. Describe two ways to insert an oral airway without pushing the tongue back.

A. _____

B. _____

36. When are oropharyngeal airways contraindicated?

37. Why is an endotracheal tube the preferred method for securing the airway during CPR?

38. Describe the proper way to ventilate during resuscitation. Include volumes, rates, ratios—all methods to avoid hyperinflation and other problems.

39. When should the endotracheal route of drug administration be used?

40. What is the primary treatment for pulseless ventricular tachycardia and ventricular fibrillation?

41. List three medications that can be delivered via the ET route.

   A. _____

   B. _____

   C. _____

42. What modification to dosage and technique must be made for endotracheal instillation of emergency drugs?

43. What initial energy level is recommended for electrical countershock during ventricular fibrillation using a biphasic defibrillator? What about monophasic? How about any subsequent shocks?

44. Explain the difference between cardioversion and defibrillation.

45. When is electrical pacing indicated?

46. Identify the drug indicated to treat each of the following. (Check out Table 34-2 in your text.)

	EVENT	**DRUG THERAPY**
A.	Ventricular tachycardia	
B.	Pulseless electrical activity	
C.	Asystole	
D.	Poor cardiac contractility	
E.	Hypotension	
F.	Hypertension	
G.	Ventricular fibrillation	
H.	SVT	
I.	Coronary artery occlusion	
J.	CHF/pulmonary edema (fluid overload)	

CASE STUDIES

Case 1

You are at a coffee shop, waiting for your coffee. A man at the corner table is eating and having coffee. Suddenly he puts his hands to his throat and tries to stand. He is unable to cough or speak.

47. What is your first action?

48. How would you remedy the FBAO?

49. If the victim becomes unconscious, how will you modify your technique?

Case 2

Your coffee is ready, but before you can drink one sip, a red-faced executive-type in a suit collapses to the floor, splashing you with dairy-free latte . . .

50. According to "Basic Life Support" guidelines, you need to perform six steps in the right order.
    A. First determine unresponsiveness. What would you check? What would you do?

    B. Step two is checking the _____,
    C. Now you need to call for help. Be specific for this setting.
    D. This victim has become unresponsive and basically dead on the spot. What device do you need right now to assess the heart and treat the most likely rhythm for sudden cardiac arrest?
    E. No devices are available. You need to start _____ at a rate of

    _____

    F. Open the _____ and check for _____.

    G. He's still dead. You should give two _____.

Case 3

You are dreaming of your coffee, but the paramedics arrive. They defibrillate the victim and his pulse returns but not his breathing. The paramedics ask for your help with airway management.

51. Select an initial device to manage the airway in an unconscious victim.

52. You must begin ventilation with bag and mask. Of course you use oxygen, but what rate is needed in this case and how long is inhalation?

53. What is the biggest hazard to the patient during bag-mask ventilation?

Circle the correct answer.

54. When is the jaw-thrust technique indicated to help maintain an airway?
    A. When foreign body obstruction is suspected
    B. In pediatric patients
    C. In cases of suspected neck injury
    D. During most CPR efforts

55. Where should you check the pulse of an unresponsive infant?
    A. Brachial artery
    B. Carotid artery
    C. Femoral artery
    D. Radial artery

56. Upon entering a hospital room, you see a physical therapist administering CPR to a patient who is lying on the

    floor. Your first action would be to _____.
    A. move the patient onto the bed
    B. call for help
    C. take over chest compressions
    D. deliver two slow breaths to the airway

57. An unconscious patient begins gagging during your attempt to insert an oropharyngeal airway. The correct action

    to take at this time would be to _____.
    A. insert a smaller oral airway
    B. intubate the patient
    C. perform the jaw-thrust maneuver
    D. insert a nasal airway

58. The ideal airway to use during a resuscitation effort is a(n) _____.
    A. oropharyngeal airway
    B. nasopharyngeal airway
    C. fenestrated tracheostomy tube
    D. oral endotracheal tube

59. A patient is coughing and wheezing after accidentally aspirating a piece of meat. At this time, the

    RT should _____.
    A. allow the patient to clear his airway
    B. perform the Heimlich maneuver
    C. deliver five back blows
    D. call for help

60. Upon entering an ICU room, an RT observes ventricular fibrillation on the cardiac monitor. The most appropriate

    treatment for this rhythm is _____.
    A. CPR
    B. administration of lidocaine
    C. administration of epinephrine
    D. defibrillation

61. During an adult resuscitation effort, no IV line can be established. The RT should recommend _____.
    A. intramuscular infusion of the medications
    B. endotracheal instillation of the medications
    C. insertion of a central line
    D. aerosol administration of the medications

62. The effectiveness of chest compressions in producing circulation can be measured by _____.
    1. pulse oximetry
    2. capnography
    3. transcutaneous monitoring
    4. arterial blood gases
       A. 1 and 2 only
       B. 2 and 3 only
       C. 2 and 4 only
       D. 1 and 4 only

63. A patient has atrial fibrillation with serious signs and symptoms that do not respond to medications. The treatment of choice would be _____.
    A. vagal stimulation
    B. defibrillation
    C. oxygen administration
    D. cardioversion

Get the picture? Any question on the subject of resuscitation is fair game. Start by learning the basic rates, depths, and management techniques. Then move on to the advanced material.

FOOD FOR THOUGHT

64. How can we improve the quality of care given during codes?

65. Who provides emotional support to the family during resuscitation of their loved one? Who provides support for the health care providers?

38 Humidity and Bland Aerosol Therapy

Define the following terms.

1. Hygrometer:

2. BTPS conditions:

3. Isothermic saturation boundary:

4. Inspissated:

MEET THE OBJECTIVES

Humidity Therapy

5. Explain inspiration and exhalation as they relate to how gas is heated and humidified under normal conditions.

6. List four factors that can shift the isothermic saturation boundary distally.

    A. _____

    B. _____

    C. _____

    D. _____

7. List four consequences of prolonged inspiration of improperly conditioned gases.

    A. _____

    B. _____

    C. _____

    D. _____

8. Liter flows exceeding what value require humidification?

9. Give one other situation where you would **ALWAYS** provide humidification.

10. List two indications for humidification.

A. _____

B. _____

11. List the four variables that affect the quality of performance of a humidifier.

A. _____

B. _____

C. _____

D. _____

Which is most important?

12. Bubble humidifiers are added to what type of oxygen delivery system?

13. What is the typical range for absolute humidity delivered by a bubble humidifier? What does this amount convert to in terms of relative body humidity?

A. Output _____ to _____ mg/L

B. Relative body humidity = _____%

14. What safety device is incorporated into the design of a bubble humidifier?

15. Discuss the three primary advantages of passover humidifiers compared with bubble humidifiers.

A. _____

B. _____

C. _____

16. Describe the principle of operation of each of the following heat and moisture exchangers (HMEs).
A. Simple condenser humidifier:

B. Hygroscopic condenser humidifier:

C. Hydrophobic condenser humidifier:

17. List five contraindications to using HMEs, according to the AARC Clinical Practice Guideline on humidification during mechanical ventilation.

A. _____

B. _____

C. _____

D. _____

E. _____

18. What is an "active HME"?

19. Identify three possible risks of using heated humidifiers.

A. _____

B. _____

C. _____

20. Identify three hazards associated with water that "rains out," or condenses, in humidified breathing circuits.

A. _____

B. _____

C. _____

21. List five factors that influence the amount of condensation in a breathing circuit.

A. _____

B. _____

C. _____

D. _____

E. _____

22. What specialized breathing circuit circumvents (usually) the condensation problem?

23. The AARC recommends what range of alarm settings for electronically controlled heated humidifiers?

Bland Aerosols

24. List seven indications given in the AARC Clinical Practice Guidelines for bland aerosol administration.

A. _____

B. _____

C. _____

D. _____

E. _____

F. _____

G. _____

25. What preset variable determines the size of the aerosol particles generated by a USN?

26. What adjustable control determines the actual amount of aerosol produced?

27. Largevolume jet nebulizers are often used to provide moisture to the airway of patients with tracheostomy tubes. When would you use this on a patient who is not intubated?

28. What provides the power to operate a largevolume jet nebulizer?

29. Large volume jet nebulizers are also useful in controlling F_IO_2. How is this accomplished?

30. Identify the two primary clinical problems associated with tents and body enclosures.

A. _____

B. _____

31. Your text identifies six important problems associated with bland aerosol therapy. For each of these problems, give a possible solution or means of prevention.

Problem	Solution
Cross-contamination/infection	_____
Environmental safety	_____
Inadequate mist	_____
Overhydration	_____
Bronchospasm	_____
Noise	_____

CALCULATIONS

32. At body temperature, gas has a saturated capacity of about 44 mg of water vapor per liter. If a gas has an absolute humidity of 22 mg/L, what is the relative humidity?

Formula _____

Solution _____

Answer _____

33. What is the humidity deficit in Question 32?

Formula _____

Solution _____

Answer _____

SUMMARY CHECKLIST

Complete the following sentences by writing the correct term(s) in the spaces provided.

34. Conditioning of _____ gases is done primarily by the _____.

35. Gases delivered to the trachea should be warmed to _____ to _____° C.

36. A _____ is a device that adds invisible molecular water to a gas.

37. A _____ generates and disperses particles into the gas stream.

38. _____ is the most important factor affecting humidifier output.

39. At high flows, some bubble humidifiers may produce _____, which can carry infectious bacteria.

40. Breathing circuit _____ must always be treated as _____ waste.

41. Bland aerosol therapy with sterile _____ is often used to treat _____ airway

_____, overcome humidity _____ in patients with tracheal airways, and help obtain

_____ specimens.

Use the algorithm in Figure 38-16 to choose the right humidity or bland aerosol system.

Case 1

A man is brought to the emergency department with a core temperature of 30° C after falling into a lake while ice fishing. The patient is intubated with a No. 8 endotracheal tube. The patient is unconscious and requires mechanical ventilation.

42. Does this patient have any contraindications for HME use?

43. What humidification system would you recommend?

Case 2

A 32-year-old man is admitted to the medical floor with a diagnosis of *Mycoplasma pneumoniae* pneumonia. He is receiving oxygen via nasal cannula at 5 L/min. He complains of a stuffy, dry nose a few hours after admission.

44. What humidification system would you recommend for this patient?

45. Why is this patient unable to benefit from an HME?

Case 3

A 57-year-old man who has undergone coronary artery bypass graft surgery (CABG) is being mechanically ventilated with a No. 8 ET tube pending recovery from the procedure. He has no secretion problems or history of lung problems. Body temperature is normal.

46. What humidification system would you recommend?

47. What signs would you see on a chest exam that would tell you that you need to switch this patient to a different device?

WHAT DOES THE NBRC SAY?

Circle the best answer.

48. A respiratory therapist hears a loud whistling sound as she enters the room of a patient receiving oxygen via cannula at 6 L/min. In reference to the humidifier, what is the most likely cause of the problem?
    A. The top of the humidifier is cross-threaded.
    B. The humidifier has run out of water.
    C. The flow rate is set at less than the ordered amount.
    D. There is a kink in the oxygen supply tubing.

49. A USN is ordered for sputum induction. Which of the following solutions should be placed in the medication cup to accomplish this goal?
    A. Sterile distilled water
    B. 0.45% NaCl solution
    C. 0.9% NaCl solution
    D. 3% NaCl solution

50. A large-volume all-purpose nebulizer is set at an F_IO_2 of 0.40 and a flow rate of 10 L/min to deliver humidified oxygen to a patient with a tracheostomy. The nebulizer is producing very little mist. Which of the following could be done to improve the aerosol output?
    1. Check the water level in the nebulizer.
    2. Increase the flow rate to the nebulizer.
    3. Drain condensate from the supply tubing.
    4. Turn off the nebulizer's heating system.
       A. 1 only
       B. 1 and 2 only
       C. 1 and 3 only
       D. 1, 3, and 4 only

51. While performing a ventilator check, the respiratory therapist observes a large amount of thin, white mucus in the tubing connected to the HME. Which of the following actions should be taken at this time?
    A. Rinse out the HME with sterile water.
    B. Suction the mucus from the tubing.
    C. Place the patient on a heated humidification system.
    D. Replace the HME.

52. Sputum induction via USN is ordered. The nebulizer will produce an output of 5 ml of water per minute on the maximum amplitude setting. The treatment is to last for 15 minutes. How much solution should the RCP respiratory therapist place in the nebulizer?
    A. 5 ml
    B. 15 ml
    C. 50 ml
    D. 75 ml

53. Which of the following patients is at greatest risk for overhydration secondary to continuous use of a heated jet nebulizer?
    A. 5-kg infant with croup
    B. 70-year-old COPD patient
    C. 25-year-old patient in need of a sputum induction
    D. 7-year-old asthma patient with pneumonia

FOOD FOR THOUGHT

54. The industry standard for adding simple humidification to an oxygen delivery system is a flow rate of greater than 4 L/min. Can you think of any situations where you might add humidification when the flow rate is lower than 4?

55. Why wouldn't you use Vapotherm or another similar system for every patient?

Chapter **38 Humidity and Bland Aerosol Therapy**

39 Aerosol Drug Therapy

WORD WIZARD

Match the following terms to their definitions.

Terms	Definitions
1. _____ Aerosol	A. Suspension of solid or liquid particles in a gas.
2. _____ Atomizer	B. Difference between therapeutic and toxic drug concentrations.
3. _____ Baffle	C. Device that produces uniformly sized aerosol particles.
4. _____ Deposition	D. Device that removes large particles.
5. _____ Hygroscopic	E. Device that produces non–uniformly sized aerosol particles.
6. _____ Inertial impaction	F. Deposition of particles by collision.
7. _____ MMAD	G. Testimony of a witness (or particles being retained in the respiratory tract!).
8. _____ Nebulizer	H. Absorbs moisture from the air.
9. _____ Propellant	I. Measurement of average particle size.
10. _____ Therapeutic index	J. Amount of drug left in the SVN.
11. _____ Residual drug volume	K. Something that provides thrust.

CHARACTERISTICS OF THERAPEUTIC AEROSOLS

12. What influence does particle size have on aerosol therapy?

13. What is the primary method of deposition for large, high-mass particles?

14. Particles of 10 microns or larger tend to be deposited in what part of the respiratory tract? What about particles between 5 and 10 microns?

   A. ≥ 10: _____

   B. 5 to 10: _____

15. In what part of the lung would you like to deposit beta-adrenergic bronchodilator medications? What particle size is needed to accomplish this goal?

   A. Where: _____

   B. Particle size: _____

16. Sedimentation is an important factor in lung deposition that RTs can influence.

    A. How long is an ideal breath hold maneuver? _____

    B. How much will you increase drug deposition? _____

    C. What about drug distribution? _____

17. It is extremely difficult to predict exactly what happens to particles once they enter the lung. What is the most practical way to determine how well you are delivering a medication?

HAZARDS OF AEROSOL THERAPY

18. Nebulizers can be a source for nosocomial infections. Describe three of the CDC's recommendations for preventing this problem.

    A. _____

    B. _____

    C. _____

19. List five aerosolized substances associated with increased airway resistance.

    A. _____

    B. _____

    C. _____

    D. _____

    E. _____

20. What can you do to help prevent bronchospasm from occurring when you nebulize reactive substances?

21. Aerosolizing drugs has the potential for inducing bronchospasm. Describe four ways you can monitor this potential problem.

    A. _____

    B. _____

    C. _____

    D. _____

22. Eye irritation is most likely to occur under what circumstances?

Metered Dose Inhalers

23. What is priming the MDI? When should it be done?

24. What other substances are found in MDIs that may produce clinical problems?

25. What percentage of the drug in an MDI is actually deposited in the lungs? Why is there so much variability?

26. List a benefit of the Aerospan.

27. Put the following steps of optimal open-mouth MDI delivery in order.

A.	Hold your breath for 10 seconds.	_____
B.	Breathe out normally.	_____
C.	Wait 1 minute.	_____
D.	Actuate canister (dose).	_____
E.	Hold the MDI two fingers from mouth.	_____
F.	Slowly inhale as deeply as you can.	_____
G.	Warm and shake the canister.	_____
H.	Actuate the canister (prime).	_____
I.	Take off the cap.	_____

28. What is the difference between a spacer and a holding chamber? Does it matter?

29. Holding chambers are especially useful for what class of inhaled medications?

30. How does the recommended breathing pattern with a holding chamber differ from that with a spacer or unassisted MDI?

Dry Powder

31. What is a DPI? How is it powered?

32. How does DPI breathing technique differ from that recommended with an MDI?

33. What patients should not use DPIs?

34. In general, what is the role of the DPI in management of acute bronchospasm?

Small Volume Nebulizers

35. List two potential power sources to drive the small volume nebulizer.

    A. _____

    B. _____

    C. _____

36. What is the ideal flow rate and amount of solution to put in an SVN for a typical albuterol treatment?

    A. Flow rate: _____

    B. Amount of solution: _____

37. What is a baffle?

38. What is meant by nebulizer "sputter," and why is it important to RTs?

39. What potential problem exists when you deliver an SVN via mask? How can you deal with this problem?

40. Explain what is meant by the "blow-by" technique used with infants and discuss the effectiveness of this technique.

41. Explain how the Respimat soft mist inhaler works.

42. You really can't nebulize all of the solution. Explain the idea of residual volume. How broad is the range?

43. What potential clinical problem may exist with continuous bronchodilator therapy?

Small Ultrasonic Nebulizers

44. List three advantages and three disadvantages of ultrasonic nebulizers (USNs) to deliver medications.

	ADVANTAGES	DISADVANTAGES
A.		
B.		
C.		

CASE STUDIES

Use the algorithms in Figure 39-33 or 39-35 in *Egan's* to answer the following questions about selection of aerosol drug delivery devices and doses.

Case 1

An alert, cooperative 52-year-old man has recently been diagnosed with chronic bronchitis. He quit smoking (60-pack-year history) 6 months ago but still has respiratory symptoms. He is in your pulmonary clinic today to receive his pulmonary function test (PFT) results and medications. The physician has ordered Atrovent and Flovent.

45. What method of delivery would you recommend for this patient?

46. What other equipment is indicated?

47. What general considerations for patient education would you stress for this patient?

48. How will you know that he is able to perform the therapy correctly?

Case 2

A 27-year-old man presents in the emergency department with acute respiratory distress. He is diagnosed with status asthmaticus. He has high-pitched diffuse wheezes, a respiratory rate of 24, a heart rate of 106, and SpO_2 of 92%. His PEFR is 150 after four puffs of albuterol via MDI.

49. What are the possible options for treating this patient at this point?

50. What method of bronchodilator delivery would you recommend?

51. What is meant by "dose-response" assessment?

Case 3

You are asked to deliver a bronchodilator to a patient in the neuro ICU. When you arrive to assess the patient, you note that she is obtunded. Breath sounds reveal scattered rhonchi and wheezing in the upper lobes.

52. What method of bronchodilator delivery would you recommend in this situation?

53. What modification will you need to make?

54. Because peak flow is unlikely to be performed, how will you assess the effectiveness of therapy?

55. What is the starting dose for albuterol via SVN for an intubated patient?

56. What standard starting dosage is recommended for albuterol by MDI to a ventilator patient?

57. Where should you place the SVN in the ventilator circuit?

58. When should an MDI be activated for a ventilator patient?

59. What adjustments to dilution need to be made with the SVN for ventilator delivery?

60. Describe the method for giving a bronchodilator to a patient on noninvasive mask ventilation.

61. Describe the method for giving a bronchodilator to a patient who is on an oscillator.

WHAT DOES THE NBRC SAY?

The following information pertains to questions 62 and 63. Circle the best answer.

Asthma has been recently diagnosed in a 16-year-old patient. The respiratory therapist is asked to teach the patient how to self-administer QVAR via MDI.

62. In addition to the inhaler, what other equipment would be needed to teach the patient?
    1. Spacer device
    2. Pulse oximeter
    3. Peak flowmeter
        A. 1 only
        B. 1 and 2 only
        C. 1 and 3 only
        D. 2 and 3 only

63. After performing the inhalation, the RT instructs the patient to perform a breath holding maneuver. The purpose of

    this maneuver is to _____.
    A. promote a strong cough
    B. improve venous return
    C. improve inertial impaction
    D. increase medication delivery

64. While attempting to administer albuterol via SVN to a patient who has had a recent CVA, the RT notes
    that the patient is unable to hold the nebulizer or keep her lips sealed on the mouthpiece. The RT should

    recommend _____.
    A. switching to an MDI
    B. utilizing an aerosol mask for delivery
    C. discontinuing the medication
    D. subcutaneous administration of the medication

65. An MDI is ordered for a patient who is intubated and being mechanically ventilated and humidified with a heat-
    moisture exchanger (HME). Which of the following is the most appropriate way to administer the bronchodilator?
    A. Place the MDI in the expiratory limb of the ventilator circuit.
    B. Place the MDI between the HME and the endotracheal tube.
    C. Recommend changing the delivery method to a small-volume nebulizer.
    D. Remove the HME during delivery of the drug.

66. An alert adult patient with asthma is receiving bronchodilator therapy via small volume nebulizer during a
    hospitalization. What should the RT do in regard to this therapy when the patient is ready for discharge?
    A. Recommend MDI instruction.
    B. Recommend oral administration of the medication.
    C. Recommend training in home use of the SVN.
    D. Recommend administration of the drug via IPPB.

67. Which of the following devices is most suitable for delivery of Tyvaso (treprostinil)?
    A. Optineb
    B. Small particle aerosol generator
    C. Ultrasonic nebulizer
    D. Atomizer

FOOD FOR THOUGHT

68. What two inhalational drugs have proved to be an occupational risk for RTs?

    A. _____

    B. _____

69. Describe some of the physical ways to control environmental contamination when delivering medications that have
    potential side effects for the provider.

70. What do the terms HEPA and PAPR refer to?

40 Storage and Delivery of Medical Gases

WORD WIZARD

Look up these nine terms and give a brief description.

Characteristics

1. Flammable _____

2. Nonflammable _____

3. Oxidizing _____

Equipment

4. Bourdon gauge _____

5. Thorpe tube _____

6. Reducing valve _____

7. Regulator _____

8. Flowmeter _____

9. Zone valves _____

CHARACTERISTICS OF MEDICAL GASES

10. List three gases that are categorized as nonflammable.

    A. _____

    B. _____

    C. _____

11. Most therapeutic gases will oxidize or support combustion. List three gases in this category.

    A. _____

    B. _____

    C. _____

12. Describe the four basic steps of the fractional distillation process.

    A. _____

    B. _____

    C. _____

    D. _____

13. What purity level is required for medical grade oxygen?

14. Describe the two methods used to separate oxygen from air. What concentration is produced by each method?

    A. _____

    B. _____

15. What is the most common use of CO_2 mixtures?

16. What is heliox? What is it used for in the clinical setting?

17. What is the primary medical use for nitrous oxide? What are some of the hazards of nitrous oxide administration?

18. Describe two possible hazards of using nitric oxide.
    A.

    B.

19. Give the chemical symbol for each of the following medical gases.

Gas	Symbol
A. Oxygen	_____
B. Air	_____
C. Carbon dioxide	_____
D. Helium	_____
E. Nitrous oxide	_____
F. Nitric oxide	_____

20. Identify the cylinder markings on the diagram shown here.

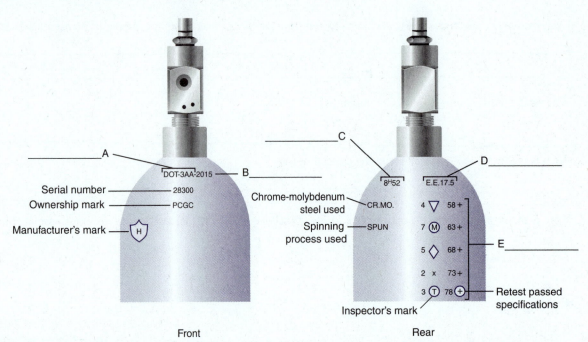

Front
Serial number — 28300
Ownership mark — PCGC
Manufacturer's mark — H

DOT-3AA-2015 — B

8H52   E.E.17.5

Rear
Chrome-molybdenum steel used — CR.MO.
Spinning process used — SPUN
Inspector's mark

4 ▽ 58 +
7 Ⓜ 63 +
5 ◇ 68 +
2 x 73 +
3 Ⓣ 78 ⊕

Retest passed specifications

These are typical markings of cylinders containing medical gases. Front and back views are for illustration purposes only. Exact location and order of markings vary.

21. What do the symbols * and + mean when stamped on a cylinder?

    A. * _____

    B. + _____

22. Identify the proper color for these gas cylinders (in the United States).

    A. Oxygen   _____

    B. Carbon dioxide _____

    C. Nitrous oxide   _____

    D. Helium   _____

    E. Nitrogen   _____

    F. Air   _____

23. Because cylinder color is only a guideline, how do you actually determine which gas is in a cylinder?

FILLING CYLINDERS

24. List two gases that can be stored in the liquid state at room temperature.

    A. _____

    B. _____

25. Explain why the pressure in a gas-filled cylinder is different from that of a liquid-filled cylinder.

26. Describe the methods for measuring the contents of a gas-filled cylinder and a liquid-filled cylinder.
    A. Gas-filled:

    B. Liquid-filled:

27. What are the cylinder factors for the "E," "G," and "H" gas-filled oxygen cylinders?
    E: _____
    G: _____
    H: _____

28. Write the formula for calculating duration of flow in minutes of gas-filled cylinders.

BULK OXYGEN

29. Describe a gaseous bulk system. Be sure to discuss the manifold, the primary, and reserve banks.

30. Why do most hospitals use a liquid bulk oxygen system?

31. Where are small liquid oxygen cylinders usually used?

32. What is the normal working pressure for a hospital oxygen piping system?

33. What are zone valves? Give two reasons you might need to use these valves.

Chapter **40 Storage and Delivery of Medical Gases**

34. If a cylinder overheats, the pressure will rise. Describe the type of pressure release valve usually found in these cylinder stems.

    Small cylinder: _____

    Large cylinder: _____

35. List the three basic indexed safety systems for medical gases. Both names!

Abbreviated name	**Full name**
A. _____	_____
B. _____	_____
C. _____	_____

36. What type of cylinder typically uses pins and holes for the safety connection system?

37. What system was established to prevent accidental interchange of low-pressure medical gas connectors? What is meant by "low-pressure"?

REGULATION PRESSURE AND FLOW

38. Describe the action of the following devices.

    A. Reducing valve: _____

    B. Flowmeter: _____

    C. Regulator: _____

39. Describe the normal way each of the following is used in respiratory care.
    A. Preset reducing valve:

    B. Adjustable reducing valve:

    C. Multiple-stage reducing valve:

40. What two hazards can be created when you open a cylinder attached to a high-pressure reducing valve?

41. What are two advantages and two disadvantages of flow restrictors?

	ADVANTAGES	DISADVANTAGES
A.		
B.		

42. Describe the Bourdon flowmeter.

43. What is the chief advantage of the Bourdon-type flowmeter?

44. What do Bourdon gauges actually measure? Thorpe tubes?

A. Bourdon: _____

B. Thorpe: _____

45. Compare indicated flow and actual flow in a compensated Thorpe flowmeter when downstream resistance occurs.

46. What happens to the float in a compensated Thorpe tube when you connect it to a 50-psi gas source?

CASE STUDY

Case 1

A patient is to be transported from the ICU to the imaging department for a CT scan. The patient requires continuous supplemental oxygen at 10 L/min by mask. You will need to provide portable oxygen for the transport. An E cylinder is available.

47. What type of regulator is most appropriate for transport?

48. How long will the cylinder last at the given flow rate if the pressure is 1000 psi?

Formula: _____

Calculation: _____

49. When you turn on the cylinder valve, a hissing noise is heard from the regulator. The flowmeter is off, so there must be a leak. What should you check to try to correct the leak?

A. _____

B. _____

MEASURING CYLINDER CONTENTS

50. Calculate duration of an E cylinder with 1500 psi running at 2 L/min.

Formula: _____

Calculation:

Answer: Minutes _____ Hours _____

51. Calculate the duration of an H cylinder with 1500 psi running at 2 L/min.

Formula: _____

Calculation:

Answer: Minutes _____ Hours _____

WHAT DOES THE NBRC SAY?

Circle the best answer.

52. An H cylinder of oxygen is being used to deliver oxygen to a patient in a subacute care facility where no piped-in oxygen is available. The cylinder gauge shows a pressure of 1000 psi. The patient is receiving oxygen at 5 L/min by cannula. Approximately how long will the cylinder gas last at this flow rate?
    A. 1 hour
    B. 8 hours
    C. 10 hours
    D. 628 hours

53. A respiratory therapist notices that a flowmeter plugged into the wall outlet continues to read 1 L/min even though it is not turned on. What is the most appropriate action at this time?
    A. Replace the flowmeter.
    B. Include the extra liter in any calculations.
    C. Disassemble the flowmeter and replace the "O-rings."
    D. Do nothing; this is not an unusual situation.

54. A respiratory therapist has to transport a patient via air from the island of Maui to Honolulu. The patient is being manually ventilated with an oxygen flow set at 10 L/min using an E cylinder of gas. The cylinder gauge reads 2000 psi. How long will the cylinder last?
    A. 42 minutes
    B. 56 minutes
    C. 60 minutes
    D. 10 hours

55. When a respiratory therapist unplugs a Thorpe-type flowmeter, a huge leak occurs from the wall outlet. What action should the RT take at this time?
    A. Shut off the gas to the room with the zone valve.
    B. Shut off the bulk oxygen system.
    C. Plug the flowmeter back into the outlet.
    D. Call maintenance to fix the outlet.

56. A fire breaks out in the pediatrics unit because of a faulty electrical cord. One respiratory therapist has ensured that patients with oxygen are safe. Your responsibility in this situation would be to
    A. prepare to shut off the zone valves to the unit.
    B. obtain an additional crash cart for emergencies.
    C. obtain additional E cylinders of oxygen.
    D. prepare to document the incident in the record.

FOOD FOR THOUGHT

57. What would happen if nitrous oxide leaked into the room in the emergency department or operating room setting?

58. Your text describes the catastrophic consequences of bulk-system failures. Describe what some of your actions might be in this type of emergency.

41 Medical Gas Therapy

OXYGEN THERAPY

Let's start by reviewing the reasons for giving oxygen and how to clinically recognize those needs.

1. What is acute hypoxemia?

2. What are the threshold criteria for defining hypoxemia in adults according to the AARC Clinical Practice Guidelines?

   1. PaO_2 _____

   2. SaO_2 _____

3. Describe the two compensatory mechanisms of the cardiopulmonary system when faced with hypoxemia.

   A. Lungs: _____

   B. Heart: _____

4. In what acute cardiac condition is oxygen therapy especially important?

5. What effect does hypoxemia have on the pulmonary blood vessels? What are the long-term consequences of this effect?

6. List three basic ways to determine when a patient needs oxygen.

   A. _____

   B. _____

   C. _____

7. List six common acute clinical situations where hypoxemia is so common that oxygen therapy is usually provided.

   A. _____

   B. _____

   C. _____

   D. _____

   E. _____

   F. _____

8. List two signs of mild and severe hypoxia for each of the following systems.

	SYSTEM	MILD	SEVERE
A.	Respiratory		
B.	Cardiovascular		
C.	Neurologic		

PRECAUTIONS AND HAZARDS OF SUPPLEMENTAL OXYGEN THERAPY

9. Oxygen toxicity can affect what two organ systems?

   A. _____

   B. _____

10. The harm caused by oxygen is influenced by what two factors?

    A. _____

    B. _____

11. Describe the effects on the lung tissue of breathing excessive oxygen.

12. What is meant by a "vicious circle" in reference to oxygen toxicity?

13. Although every patient is unique, what general rule of thumb can be applied to prevent oxygen toxicity?

14. What specific type of COPD patient is likely to experience depression of ventilatory drive while breathing oxygen?

15. When should oxygen be withheld from a hypoxic COPD patient to avoid depressing ventilation?

16. During what time period after birth is a preemie likely to develop ROP?

17. How can you reduce the risk of ROP?

18. Describe how oxygen can cause atelectasis.

19. How can you reduce the risk of absorption atelectasis?

20. What is the fire triangle?

21. What is the biggest hazard in the home setting?

OXYGEN DELIVERY SYSTEMS

22. The three basic categories of oxygen delivery systems are low flow, high flow, and reservoir. Match the category to the description below.

	CATEGORY	DESCRIPTION
A.	Low flow	Always exceeds patient's inspiratory needs
B.	Reservoir	Provides some of patient's inspiratory needs
C.	High flow	May meet needs if no leaks occur

LOW FLOW

23. When should you attach the cannula to a bubble humidifier?

24. What maximum flow does the text suggest for newborns?

25. How does the patient's breathing pattern affect the F_1O_2 delivered to the lungs when using a low-flow device such as a cannula?

26. What is the primary disadvantage of the transtracheal catheter?

27. What range of F_1O_2 is usually delivered by low-flow devices?

28. Because you can't tell exactly how much oxygen the patient is receiving at any given moment from a cannula or any low-flow device, how can you assess the effects of administering the drug?

29. In what setting are reservoir cannulas usually used?

30. Use Table 41-3 to help you find the information about oxygen masks.

	MASK	F_IO_2 RANGE	ADVANTAGE	DISADVANTAGE
A.	Simple			
B.	Partial rebreathing			
C.	Nonrebreathing			

31. What is the primary difference between the partial rebreathing and nonrebreathing masks?

32. How can you tell if a nonrebreathing mask has an adequate flow rate?

33. Give a solution for each of these common problems with reservoir masks.

	Problem	**Solution**
A.	No gas felt from cannula	_____
B.	Humidifier pop-off activated	_____
C.	Mask causes claustrophobia	_____
D.	Bag collapses on inspiration	_____
E.	Bag fully inflated on inspiration	_____

HIGH FLOW

34. Describe the effects of varying the jet size or entrainment port opening on F_IO_2 and total flow rate.

	FACTOR	INCREASED SIZE	DECREASED SIZE
A.	Jet 1. F_IO_2 2. Flow		
B.	Port 1. F_IO_2 2. Flow		

35. Fill in the air-to-oxygen ratios for the following oxygen concentrations.

A. 100% _____

B. 60% _____

C. 40% _____

D. 35% _____

E. 30% _____

F. 24% _____

36. Why does the AEM have larger openings on the side of the mask than a simple oxygen mask?

37. What effect does raising the delivered flow from the flowmeter have on the F_IO_2 delivered by an AEM?

38. How do you boost the total flow when using an AEM?

39. There are four devices used to deliver gas from an air-entrainment nebulizer to the patient. Choose the device(s) that fits each of the following patients. (See Figure 41-16 in your text.)

Patient	Aerosol Delivery Device
A. Tracheostomy tube	_____
B. Endotracheal tube	_____
C. Intact upper airway	_____
D. After nasal surgery	_____

40. Describe an easy way to tell if an air-entrainment nebulizer is providing sufficient gas to meet the patient's needs.

41. Give one example of a specialized flow generator that produces an aerosol.

42. What effect does downstream resistance to flow have on F_IO_2 and total flow delivered by a typical AEM or nebulizer entrainment system?

43. What is the oxygen to air entrainment ratio and total flow for a patient who is receiving 60% oxygen via an entrainment nebulizer with the flowmeter set at 10 L/min?

A. Step 1: Compute the ratio.

Formula: _____

Calculation: _____

Reduce answer to get ratio: _____

B. Step 2: Add the parts.

C. Step 3: Multiply the sum of the parts by the O₂ flow rate.

BLENDERS AND HOODS

44. Describe the three-step process for confirming the proper operation of a blender.

A. _____

B. _____

C. _____

45. Why is a hood the best method for delivering oxygen to an infant?

46. What minimum flow must be set for a hood? Why?

47. What harmful consequence occurs when flow rates into the hood are too high?

48. What effect will cold air flowing into the hood have on a premature infant?

49. What is the best way to control oxygen delivery to an infant inside an incubator?

50. What is the primary benefit of the infant incubator?

HIGH-FLOW SYSTEMS AND HYPOXEMIA

High-flow oxygen systems are a valuable new tool for managing serious hypoxemia.

51. What three main features make the Vapotherm and Fisher and Paykel's Optiflow high-flow systems useful in treating moderate hypoxemia?

52. What are the major limitations of these devices?

53. What device could you use during resuscitation or in the emergency setting to administer 100% oxygen?

HYPERBARIC OXYGEN

54. Compare the monoplace and multiplace hyperbaric chambers.

	CHAMBER	O_2 DELIVERY	PATIENT	STAFF
A.	Monoplace			
B.	Multiplace			

55. List three acute and three chronic conditions in which HBO is indicated. (See Box 41-6.)

Acute   Chronic

A. _____   _____

B. _____   _____

C. _____   _____

56. Under what circumstances is HBO indicated in cases of carbon monoxide poisoning?

OTHER GASES

57. Two other therapeutic gases are commonly administered by RTs. Give indications for each.

Gas	Indications
A. NO	_____
	_____
B. Helium	_____
	_____

58. What other gas is always mixed with helium? What is the most common combination?

59. What physical property of helium results in decreased work of breathing?

CASE STUDIES

Case 1

A 52-year-old college professor is admitted for chest pain and possible myocardial infarction (MI). Electrocardiogram (ECG) monitoring reveals sinus tachycardia. The chest pain has been decreased by the administration of nitroglycerin. Respirations are 20 per minute, and SpO_2 on room air is 92%.

60. What is your assessment of this patient's oxygenation status?

61. What is your recommendation in regard to administration of supplemental oxygen?

A man has been admitted for exacerbation of his COPD. The patient is receiving oxygen at 2 L/min via nasal cannula. The pulse oximeter shows a saturation of 94% while at rest. The nurse calls you to ask for your assistance in evaluation of the patient's dyspnea during ambulation.

62. What changes occur in breathing pattern during exercise?

63. How are low-flow oxygen devices affected by changes in breathing pattern?

64. How would you assess dyspnea on ambulation for a patient wearing oxygen?

A patient is recovering from surgery following a head injury. The patient is trached and requires supplemental oxygen at 60% via T-piece. The flowmeter is set at 12 L/min. Each time the patient inhales, the mist exiting the T-piece disappears.

65. Air-entrainment nebulizers are considered high-flow delivery systems. Discuss this in terms of the disappearing mist.

66. What should be added to the T-piece to help deal with this problem?

67. Describe a common method of increasing the delivered flow when administering high F_iO_2 via air-entrainment nebulizers.

68. What is the oxygen to air entrainment ratio for 60%?

69. What is the total flow in the system described in this case?

Circle the best answer.

70. During a suctioning procedure a patient experiences tachycardia with PVCs. Which of the following could be responsible for this response?
    A. Inadequate vacuum pressure
    B. Lack of sterile technique during the procedure
    C. Fear of the suctioning procedure
    D. Inadequate preoxygenation

71. A patient with a history of carbon dioxide retention is receiving oxygen at 6 L/min via nasal cannula. He is becoming lethargic and difficult to arouse. In regard to the oxygen delivery, what change would you recommend?
    A. Change to a 40% Venturi mask.
    B. Maintain the present therapy.
    C. Change to a partial rebreathing mask.
    D. Reduce the flow to 2 L/min and obtain an ABG.

72. A newborn requires oxygen therapy. Which of the following methods of delivery would you select?
    A. Partial rebreathing mask
    B. Oxygen hood
    C. Venturi mask
    D. Oxygen tent

73. A patient is receiving oxygen therapy from a nonrebreathing mask with a flow rate of 10 L/min. The respiratory therapist observes the bag deflating with each inspiration. What action is indicated in this situation?
    A. Replace the mask with a cannula.
    B. Immediately perform pulse oximetry.
    C. Increase the flow to the mask.
    D. Change to a Venturi mask.

74. A patient is to receive a mixture of helium and oxygen. Which of the following delivery devices would be appropriate?
    A. Nasal cannula
    B. Oxygen tent
    C. Venturi mask
    D. Nonrebreathing mask

75. An 80/20 mixture of helium and oxygen is administered. An oxygen flowmeter is set at 10 L/min. What is the actual flow delivered to the patient?
    A. 10 L
    B. 14 L
    C. 16 L
    D. 18 L

76. A patient is receiving 40% oxygen via an air-entrainment mask with the flowmeter set at 8 L/min. What is the total flow delivered to the patient?
    A. 24 L/min
    B. 32 L/min
    C. 40 L/min
    D. 48 L/min

77. A patient requires a flow rate of 40 L/min to meet his inspiratory demand for gas. He is to receive oxygen via a Venturi mask set at 24%. What is the minimum setting on the flowmeter to produce the appropriate flow?
    A. 1 L/min
    B. 2 L/min
    C. 3 L/min
    D. 4 L/min

78. Why does common use of the term "100% nonrebreather" create a clinical problem?

79. Why would an AEM be preferred over an air-entrainment nebulizer for a patient who has asthma or COPD?

42 Lung Expansion Therapy

WORD WIZARD

For each of the following terms or treatments, give a simple, short explanation in lay terms that your patient could understand.

1. Atelectasis: "When you don't take deep breaths . . ."

2. Incentive spirometer (IS):
   A. "The purpose of this treatment is to . . ."

   _____

   B. "This device will . . ."

   _____

3. Sustained maximal inspiration (SMI): "I want you to take . . ."

4. Continuous positive airway pressure (CPAP)
   A. "This treatment will . . ."

   _____

   B. "I am going to put a mask on your face . . ."

   _____

MEET THE OBJECTIVES

Answer the following questions to test your understanding of this chapter's objectives.

5. What is the definition of atelectasis?

6. What is resorption atelectasis, and when is it likely to occur?

7. What causes compression atelectasis?

8. Why are postoperative patients at highest risk for development of atelectasis?

9. Which specific group of postoperative patients is at highest risk of developing atelectasis?

10. List two other types of patients who have increased likelihood of developing atelectasis. Explain why.
    A. _____
    B. _____

11. Explain how each of the following may help provide clues that atelectasis is present or likely.
    A. History

    B. Breath sounds

    C. Respiratory rate

    D. Heart rate

    E. Chest radiography

12. List three indications, two contraindications, and two hazards of incentive spirometry.
    A. Indications

    1. _____

    2. _____

    3. _____

    B. Contraindications

    1. _____

    2. _____

    C. Hazards

    1. _____

    2. _____

13. Consider the complications of hyperventilation and pain. What are your ideas about dealing with these problems?
    A. Hyperventilation:

    B. Pain:

14. Give a brief general idea of how intermittent positive airway pressure breathing (IPPB) works to inflate the lung when the patient cannot take a deep breath.

15. Like IS, IPPB is used to treat atelectasis. Specifically, when would IPPB be indicated compared with IS?

16. List five contraindications to IPPB.

    A. _____

    B. _____

    C. _____

    D. _____

    E. _____

302

17. List two common complications of IPPB administration.

    A. _____

    B. _____

18. List three current positive airway pressure (PAP) therapies.

    A. _____

    B. _____

    C. _____

19. List four factors that contribute to the benefit of PEP, flutter, and CPAP.

    A. _____

    B. _____

    C. _____

    D. _____

20. List two contraindications to CPAP therapy.

    A. _____

    B. _____

21. What alarm system is essential for monitoring patients receiving continuous mask CPAP?

22. List three complications of prolonged bed rest. How would you remedy this problem?

    A. _____

    B. _____

    C. _____

    Remedy:

SUMMARY CHECKLIST

Complete the following sentences by writing the correct term(s) in the spaces provided.

23. Atelectasis is caused by persistent _____ with _____ tidal volumes.

24. Patients who have undergone upper _____ or _____ surgery are at the greatest risk for atelectasis.

25. A history of _____ disease or _____ are additional risk factors.

26. The chest _____ is often used to confirm the presence of atelectasis.

27. Patients with atelectasis usually demonstrate _____ breathing.

28. The most common problem associated with lung expansion therapy is the onset of respiratory _____, which occurs when the patient breathes _____.

CASE STUDIES

Use the protocol found in Figure 42-8 and the section on "selecting an approach" to help answer the following questions.

Case 1

An alert 34-year-old man is admitted for a hernia repair. He smokes two packs of cigarettes per day. Following surgery, the physician asks for your recommendation for therapy to prevent lung complications. The patient's vital capacity is 1.4 L, and he weighs 80 kg, his ideal body weight. He complains of cough but produces no sputum.

29. Discuss potential risk factors for atelectasis in this case.

30. What therapy would you recommend for prevention of atelectasis for this patient?

Case 2

A 70-year-old, 5-foot 2-inch female patient is immobilized following hip replacement. Her predicted inspiratory capacity is 1.8 L. She is performing incentive spirometry at 500 ml per breath. Breath sounds reveal bilateral basilar crackles, and she is coughing up lots of thick mucus.

31. What is the minimum acceptable volume for incentive spirometry for this patient according to her predicted IC and her measured volume?

32. What treatment would you recommend adding to the therapeutic regimen at this time?

WHAT DOES THE NBRC SAY?

Circle the best answer.

33. A patient complains of a "tingling" feeling in her lips during an incentive spirometry treatment. The RT should

    instruct the patient to _____.
    A. breathe more slowly
    B. take smaller breaths
    C. continue with the treatment as ordered
    D. exhale through pursed lips after each breath

34. Which of the following alarms is a vital part of the system when setting up CPAP therapy for treatment of atelectasis?
    A. Exhaled volume
    B. High respiratory rate
    C. Pulse oximetry
    D. Low pressure

35. During administration of IPPB therapy, the practitioner observes the system pressure rise suddenly at the end of

    inspiration. The RT should instruct the patient to _____
    A. "Help the machine give you a deep breath."
    B. "Inhale slowly along with the machine."
    C. "Exhale gently and normally."
    D. "Exhale through pursed lips after each breath."

36. A patient is having difficulty initiating each breath with an IPPB machine. The practitioner should adjust the

    _____.
    A. pressure limit
    B. peak flow
    C. F_iO_2
    D. sensitivity

37. Which control is used to increase the volume delivered by an IPPB machine?
    A. Pressure limit
    B. Peak flow
    C. F_iO_2
    D. Sensitivity

38. Continuous positive airway pressure is used to increase which of the following?
    A. Functional residual capacity
    B. Peak expiratory flow rate
    C. FEV_1
    D. Arterial carbon dioxide levels

39. An IPPB machine cycles on with the patient effort but does not shut off. The most likely cause of this problem is

    _____.
    A. the pressure is set too low
    B. the sensitivity is set incorrectly
    C. there is a leak in the system
    D. the patient is not blowing out hard enough

40. How should you instruct a patient to breathe during incentive spirometry?
    A. "Exhale gently, then inhale rapidly through the spirometer."
    B. "Inhale deeply and rapidly through the spirometer."
    C. "Exhale until your lungs are empty, then inhale and hold your breath."
    D. "Exhale normally, then inhale slowly and deeply and hold your breath."

41. How often should a patient be instructed to use the incentive spirometer after being taught to perform the procedure correctly?
    A. 10 breaths, four times per day
    B. 6 to 10 breaths every hour
    C. 10 to 20 breaths every 2 hours
    D. 6 to 8 breaths three times daily

42. A patient who has had surgery for an abdominal aortic aneurysm suffers from arrhythmias and hypotension after surgery. The physician asks for your recommendation for lung expansion therapy. The best choice in this situation

would be _____.
A. IS
B. IPPB
C. PEP
D. CPAP

43. When adjusting the flow rate control on an IPPB machine, the RT would be altering the _____.
A. maximum pressure delivered by the device
B. effort required to initiate a breath
C. volume delivered by the machine
D. inspiratory time for a given breath

FOOD FOR THOUGHT

44. A really interesting topic in critical care is how best to reinflate the acutely restricted or atelectatic lung. "Lung recruitment maneuvers" is the correct name. Why don't you search this and explain briefly, in your own terms, how a lung recruitment maneuver is done.

43 Airway Clearance Therapy (ACT)

Write out each of these acronyms.

1. ACBT _____
2. PEP _____
3. AD _____
4. PDPV _____
5. CPT _____
6. CPAP _____
7. EPAP _____
8. FET _____
9. HFCWC _____
10. HZ _____
11. ICP _____
12. IPV _____
13. MI-E _____

AIRWAY CLEARANCE

14. List the four phases of the normal cough. Give examples of impairments for each.

Phase	**Impairments**
A. _____	_____
B. _____	_____
C. _____	_____
D. _____	_____

15. Compare the effects of full and partial airway obstruction caused by retained secretions.

A. Full obstruction, or _____ plugging, results in _____.

B. Partial obstruction increases _____ of breathing and leads to air _____.

DISEASE AND BAD CLEARANCE

16. List three conditions that may cause internal obstruction or external compression of the airway lumen.

    A. _____

    B. _____

    C. _____

17. List two obstructive lung diseases that result in excessive secretion of mucus and impairment of normal clearance.

    A. _____

    B. _____

18. List four neurologic or musculoskeletal conditions that impair cough.

    A. _____

    B. _____

    C. _____

    D. _____

SECRETION MANAGEMENT: GOALS AND INDICATIONS

19. List four acute conditions in which bronchial hygiene is indicated.

    A. _____

    B. _____

    C. _____

    D. _____

20. Discuss bronchial hygiene therapy for chronic lung conditions. How much sputum needs to be produced daily for the therapy to be useful? What are three typical diseases that we treat?

21. Describe the two well-documented preventive, or prophylactic, uses of bronchial hygiene therapy.
    A.

    B.

22. Give a brief explanation of the significance of each factor listed below.

Factor	Significance
A. History	_____
B. Airway	_____
C. Chest radiograph	_____
D. Breath sounds	_____
E. Vital signs	_____

BRONCHIAL HYGIENE METHODS

23. Postural drainage therapy includes up to four components, not counting cough. What are they?

A. _____

B. _____

C. _____

D. _____

24. List two absolute and two relative contraindications to turning.
    A. Absolute

    1. _____

    2. _____

    B. Relative

    1. _____

    2. _____

25. How long should you wait to schedule postural drainage after a patient eats? Why?

26. What is the minimum range of time for effective application of postural drainage therapy?

27. Give a recommended intervention for each of the complications of postural drainage listed below.

Complication	Interventions
A. Hypoxemia	_____
B. Increased ICP	_____
C. Acute hypotension	_____
D. Pulmonary bleeding	_____
E. Vomiting	_____
F. Bronchospasm	_____
G. Cardiac dysrhythmias	_____

28. How long does it take to determine the effectiveness of postural drainage? If therapy is effective, how often should you reevaluate in the hospital? In the home?

   A. How long? _____

   B. Reevaluate hospital patients? _____

   C. Reevaluate home patients? _____

29. List five factors that must be documented after each postural drainage treatment:

   A. _____

   B. _____

   C. _____

   D. _____

   E. _____

30. Describe percussion and vibration as techniques to loosen secretions. Are they really effective?

31. Compare manual and mechanical methods of percussion and vibration.

Coughing and Related Expulsion Techniques

32. How would you position a patient (ideally) for an effective cough?

33. Standard directed cough must frequently be modified. Give three examples of types of patients who may need modified cough techniques.

   A. _____

   B. _____

   C. _____

34. What is splinting?

35. What special form of cough assistance is used with patients who have neuromuscular conditions?

310

36. Describe the forced expiratory technique (FET).

37. Describe the three repeated cycles of the ACB technique.

    A. _____

    B. _____

    C. _____

38. What is the primary problem with autogenic drainage?

39. Describe the two cycles of MI-E in terms of time and pressure.
    A. Inspiratory:

    B. Expiratory:

Positive Airway Pressure

40. Positive airway pressure is a popular way to help mobilize secretions. What are the four indications for PAP adjuncts according to the AARC Clinical Practice Guidelines?

    A. _____

    B. _____

    C. _____

    D. _____

41. What type of monitoring is essential regardless of the equipment used to deliver positive airway pressure to help mobilize secretions?

High-Frequency Compression/Oscillation of the Chest Wall

42. Describe the two general approaches to oscillation.

    A. _____

    B. _____

43. Describe the way IPV delivers gas to the airway.

44. Describe four of the benefits or advantages of the flutter valve as a secretion management tool.

    A. _____

    B. _____

    C. _____

    D. _____

Mobilization and Exercise

45. Describe the benefits of adding exercise as a mobilization technique.

46. What should you specifically monitor when exercising patients with lung problems?

CASE STUDIES

Case 1

Refer to Figure 40-12 for some clues.

A 60-year-old professor who has had a colon resection for an intestinal tumor is receiving incentive spirometry to help expand his lungs. You are asked to assess the patient for retained secretions. Auscultation reveals coarse rhonchi bilaterally in the upper lobes. A few scattered crackles are heard in the bases. SpO_2 on room air is 94%. The patient states he is unable to cough up anything "because it hurts too much."

47. What technique could you use to decrease the pain associated with cough in a postoperative patient?

48. What type of cough would you teach this patient?

A 75-year-old woman with bronchiectasis states she coughs up "cups of awful mucus every day." She is admitted with a diagnosis of pneumonia.

49. What therapy is indicated while this patient is in the hospital?

    As you provide the therapy, you find out that the patient is a widow who lives alone. She takes albuterol treatments via SVN when she has difficulty breathing.

50. What therapy alternatives could you recommend for home use?

WHAT DOES THE NBRC SAY?

Circle the best answer.

51. During the initial treatment, a PEP device is set to deliver a pressure of 15 cm H_2O. The patient complains of dyspnea and can maintain exhalation only for a short period of time. Which of the following should the RT recommend?
    A. Decrease the PEP level to 10 cm H_2O.
    B. Increase the PEP level to 20 cm H_2O.
    C. Discontinue the PEP therapy.
    D. Add a bronchodilator to the PEP therapy.

52. A patient is lying on her left side, turned one-quarter toward her back, with the head of the bed down. What division of the lung is being drained?
    A. Lateral segments of the right lower lobe
    B. Right middle lobe
    C. Left upper lobe, lingular segments
    D. Posterior segment of the right upper lobe

53. A patient is receiving postural drainage in the Trendelenburg position. The patient begins to cough uncontrollably. What action should the RT take at this time?
    A. Encourage the patient to use a huff cough.
    B. Administer oxygen therapy.
    C. Administer a bronchodilator.
    D. Raise the head of the bed.

54. In explaining the therapeutic goal of PEP therapy to a patient, it would be most appropriate to say:
    A. "This will help prevent pneumonia."
    B. "This will increase your intrathoracic pressure."
    C. "This will help you cough more effectively."
    D. "This will prevent atelectasis."

55. A COPD patient with left lower lobe infiltrates is unable to tolerate a head-down position for postural drainage. What action would you recommend?
    A. Perform the drainage with the head of the bed raised.
    B. Do not perform the therapy until 2 hours after the last meal.
    C. Administer a bronchodilator prior to the postural drainage.
    D. Notify the physician and suggest a different secretion management technique.

56. Active patient participation is an important part of which of the following procedures?
    1. Postural drainage
    2. Directed cough techniques
    3. Airway suctioning
    4. Positive expiratory pressure (PEP)
       A. 1 and 2 only
       B. 2 and 4 only
       C. 1 and 3 only
       D. 3 and 4 only

57. An RT is preparing a patient with bronchiectasis for discharge. Which of the following techniques would be most appropriate for self-administered therapy in the home?
    A. IPPB
    B. Flutter
    C. Suctioning
    D. Percussion and postural drainage

FOOD FOR THOUGHT

58. How does hydration affect secretion clearance? What respiratory therapy modality can augment hydration of the airway?

59. Your text mentions never clapping directly over the spine or clavicles. Can you think of other areas you should not clap over?

44 Respiratory Failure and the Need for Ventilatory Support

WORD WIZARD

Match the definitions to these seven concepts.

_____ Auto-PEEP

_____ Barotrauma

_____ Dynamic hyperinflation

_____ Type I respiratory failure

_____ Type II respiratory failure

_____ Respiratory alternans

_____ Work of breathing

A. Switching from abdominal to ribcage breathing.
B. Another term for dynamic hyperinflation.
C. The oxygen is too low.
D. The carbon dioxide is too high.
E. The physiologic cost of increased dead space and resistance.
F. Hyperinflation, elevated airway pressures, and procedures lead to this harmful outcome.
G. Low rates, high flows, and moderate volumes avoid this harmful outcome.

RESPIRATORY FAILURE

1. Complete this sentence: "Put simply, respiratory failure is the _____."

2. Define the blood gas criteria for respiratory failure.

   A. PaO_2: _____

   B. $PaCO_2$: _____

3. What are the two general types of respiratory failure based on the type of physiologic impairment?

   A. Type I: _____

   B. Type II: _____

4. Give an example of an arterial blood gas presentation of acute hypoxemic respiratory failure due to $\dot{V}/\dot{Q}$ mismatch or shunt.

5. What is the relationship between $PaCO_2$ and alveolar ventilation?

315

6. Give two examples of specific disorders responsible for acute hypercapnic respiratory failure (Type II).
A. Decreased ventilatory drive

1. _____

2. _____

B. Respiratory muscle fatigue/failure

1. _____

2. _____

C. Increased work of breathing

1. _____

2. _____

7. Give an example of a condition that could cause greatly increased CO_2 production.

ACUTE-ON-CHRONIC RESPIRATORY FAILURE

8. How does the body compensate for chronically elevated carbon dioxide levels associated with COPD or obesity hypoventilation syndrome?

9. Describe what happens to the normal blood gas classification of respiratory failure in patients with chronic respiratory failure.

10. Identify five of the most common precipitating factors that lead to acute-on-chronic failure.

A. _____

B. _____

C. _____

D. _____

E. _____

11. List four treatment goals for this group of patients.

A. _____

B. _____

C. _____

D. _____

12. Identify the likely causes of pulmonary complications from treating acute respiratory failure.

A. Emboli _____

B. Barotrauma _____

C. Infection _____

13. Give one example of each of these nonpulmonary complications of life in the ICU.

A. Cardiac _____

B. Gastrointestinal _____

C. Renal _____

INDICATIONS FOR VENTILATORY SUPPORT

14. What is the goal of mechanical ventilation?

15. Fill in the following table regarding the physiologic indicators for ventilatory support.

Mechanism	Normal and Critical Values
A. $PaCO_2$	_____
B. pH	_____
C. VC (ml/kg)	_____
D. MIP	_____
E. MVV	_____
F. V_E	_____
G. V_D/V_T	_____
H. $P(A - a)O_2$ on 100%	_____
I. P/F ratio	_____

16. What P/F ratio is considered an indicator of profoundly impaired oxygenation?

17. Why is it useful to consider pH when evaluating carbon dioxide levels to determine the need to intubate and ventilate a patient?

Chapter **44** **Respiratory Failure and the Need for Ventilatory Support**

18. Define "MIP" and give the minimal value for most patients.

    A. _____

    B. _____

19. What patient group is most likely to develop respiratory muscle weakness?

20. List three conditions that frequently lead to respiratory muscle fatigue.

    A. _____

    B. _____

    C. _____

STRATEGIES

21. Define noninvasive ventilation.

22. NIV can blow off the CO_2 and improve the Os via several mechanisms. List three of them.

    A. _____

    B. _____

    C. _____

23. NIV is useful for treating COPD with respiratory failure. State two benefits of this therapy.

    A. When is NIV useful for COPD?

    B. When is it less effective?

    C. Do COPD patients actually tolerate this procedure?

24. What cardiac condition is also treated by NIV?

25. Is NIV useful for treating ARDS? What does the evidence show?

26. Why is NIV unlikely to help with obesity hypoventilation syndrome?

INVASIVE VENTILATORY SUPPORT

27. List the three variables you will set in volume ventilation.

   A. _____

   B. _____

   C. _____

28. Name the three set variables in pressure ventilation.

   A. _____

   B. _____

   C. _____

29. What two variables are always set by the operator regardless of volume or pressure modes?

   A. _____

   B. _____

SPECIAL CASES

30. What is the main strategy for reducing lung injury in ARDS according to Chapter 44?

31. How does hyperventilation result in reduced ICP in head injury? What is the target $PaCO_2$ in these cases?

32. What is the chief concern regarding use of PEEP to increase oxygenation in patients with acute head injuries?

33. Air-trapping, or hyperinflation, as a result of obstructive lung disease causes what two complications in mechanically ventilated patients?

A. _____

B. _____

34. How are tidal volume and flow rate manipulated to reduce complications in mechanically ventilated COPD patients?

A. Tidal volume _____

B. Flow rate _____

35. What surprising technique was found to reduce auto-PEEP?

36. What is the specific goal in regard to CO_2 in respiratory failure in the chronic hypercapnic patient with COPD?

SUMMARY CHECKLIST

Complete the following sentences by writing the correct term(s) in the spaces provided.

37. Acute respiratory failure is identified by a $PaCO_2$ of greater than _____ mm Hg and/or a PaO_2 of less than _____ mm Hg in an otherwise healthy individual (at sea level, of course).

38. _____ respiratory failure is usually due to $\dot{V}/\dot{Q}$ mismatch or intrapulmonary _____, or

_____.

39. Chronic respiratory failure may be represented by ABGs demonstrating _____ with evidence of

metabolic compensation or _____ reflecting chronic hypoxemia.

40. Excessive _____ is the most common cause of respiratory muscle fatigue.

41. Only patients with rapidly reversible conditions should undergo _____ ventilation in the acute setting.

42. The goal of therapy in acute hypercapnic respiratory failure is to guarantee a set _____ ventilation.

Case 1

An alert, anxious 25-year-old woman presents in the emergency department complaining of chills, fever, and shortness of breath. An arterial blood gas is drawn on room air with these results:

pH	7.45
$PaCO_2$	32 mm Hg
PaO_2	50 mm Hg
HCO_3^-	23 mEq/L

43. Interpret this blood gas.

44. What is the A-a gradient?

45. What type of respiratory failure is present?

46. What do you recommend for initial respiratory treatment?

Case 2

A 27-year-old is brought to the emergency department by paramedics following a drug overdose. The patient is obtunded. Blood gases are drawn on room air:

pH	7.24
$PaCO_2$	60 mm Hg
PaO_2	65 mm Hg
HCO_3^-	26 mEq/L

47. Interpret this blood gas.

48. What is the A-a gradient?

49. What type of respiratory failure is present?

50. What is the appropriate initial respiratory treatment in this case?

An alert 56-year-old man with a history of COPD presents in the emergency department complaining of dyspnea, which has worsened over the last few days. A blood gas is drawn on room air:

pH	7.26
$PaCO_2$	70 mm Hg
PaO_2	50 mm Hg
HCO_3^-	32 mEq/L

51. Interpret this blood gas.

52. What is the A-a gradient?

53. What type of respiratory failure is present?

54. What initial respiratory treatments are indicated? What are we trying to avoid?

WHAT DOES THE NBRC SAY?

Circle the best answer.

55. An RT is asked to evaluate a lethargic 50-year-old woman who is in respiratory distress following abdominal surgery. She is breathing spontaneously on a 50% air-entrainment mask at 32 breaths per minute. ABG results show:

pH	7.28
$PaCO_2$	55 mm Hg
PaO_2	60 mm Hg
HCO_3^-	26 mEq/L

Based on this information, what would you recommend?
A. Provide intubation and mechanical ventilation.
B. Increase the F_IO_2 to 1.0.
C. Administer CPAP.
D. Administer bronchodilator therapy via SVN.

56. An alert, anxious 60-year-old man with a history of CHF presents in the ED with respiratory distress. Auscultation reveals bilateral inspiratory crackles. He has peripheral edema. ABG results drawn on a partial rebreathing mask show:

pH	7.45
$PaCO_2$	35 mm Hg
PaO_2	40 mm Hg
HCO_3^-	23 mEq/L

The most appropriate therapy for improving oxygenation would be to
A. provide intubation and mechanical ventilation.
B. administer oxygen therapy via nonrebreathing mask.
C. administer oxygen therapy via CPAP.
D. administer bronchodilator therapy via SVN.

57. An adult patient is being mechanically ventilated following respiratory failure. Settings are:

Tidal volume	600 ml
Rate	12
Mode	AC/VC
F_iO_2	0.60
PEEP	3 cm H_2O

ABGs show:

pH	7.37
$PaCO_2$	41 mm Hg
PaO_2	43 mm Hg
HCO_3^-	22 mEq/L

Which of the following ventilator changes would you recommend at this time?
A. Increase the F_iO_2.
B. Decrease the volume.
C. Increase the rate.
D. Increase the PEEP.

58. A patient with a history of hypercapnia and COPD is intubated and placed on the ventilator following respiratory failure. 24 hours later, the patient is alert and breathing spontaneously. Settings are:

Tidal volume	650 ml
Rate	12
Mode	AC/VC
F_iO_2	0.30
PEEP	0 cm H_2O

ABGs show:

pH	7.48
$PaCO_2$	41 mm Hg
PaO_2	60 mm Hg
HCO_3^-	30 mEq/L

Which of the following ventilator changes would you recommend at this time?
A. Decrease the F_iO_2.
B. Decrease the volume.
C. Change to pressure-controlled ventilation (PCV).
D. Change to continuous positive airway pressure (CPAP).

59. A 77-year-old man with COPD is admitted with acute bronchitis. Room air blood gas results show:

pH	7.52
$PaCO_2$	45 mm Hg
PaO_2	50 mm Hg
HCO_3^-	36 mEq/L

What intervention would be appropriate at this time?
A. CPAP with 24% oxygen
B. 28% Air entrainment mask
C. Nasal cannula at 5 L/min
D. Simple mask at 8 L/min

FOOD FOR THOUGHT

60. What clinical situations or conditions suggest using ABGs to evaluate the need to intubate and ventilate? Compare this with situations better assessed by measures such as VC and MIP.

45 Mechanical Ventilators

WORD WIZARD

Match these definitions to the key terms.

Definitions	Terms
1. _____ Breath initiated by the ventilator.	A. Spontaneous breath
2. _____ Causes a breath to end.	B. Control variable
3. _____ Manipulated by machine to cause inspiration.	C. Limit variable
4. _____ Controls the magnitude of inspiration.	D. Cycle variable
5. _____ Combination of machine and spontaneous breaths.	E. Intermittent mandatory ventilation
6. _____ Machine breaths only—no spontaneous breaths.	F. Trigger variable
7. _____ Spontaneous breaths only—no machine breaths.	G. CMV
8. _____ Causes a breath to begin.	H. CSV
9. _____ Breath initiated and ended by the patient.	I. Mandatory breath

HOW VENTILATORS WORK

10. What is a ventilator?

11. Describe the desired output of the ventilator in terms of the patient.

12. Identify two settings where ventilators can use rechargeable battery power sources.

    A. _____

    B. _____

13. How are most modern intensive care ventilators powered?

14. What does the output control valve do?

A. Regulates: _____

B. Shapes: _____

15. How do electrical circuits control ventilator operations?

VENTILATOR DISPLAYS AND ALARM SETTINGS

16. List four ways monitored data can be displayed. Give an example of each.

A. _____

B. _____

C. _____

D. _____

17. What is the purpose of a ventilator alarm?

18. What is an event? Explain the levels of priority with an example of each.
Event:

Level 1: _____

Level 2: _____

Level 3: _____

Level 4: _____

19. How do ventilators display alarms? Does this present any problems?

20. What two factors can cause pressure, volume, and flow to differ from the set values to the output values?

A. _____

B. _____

IDENTIFYING MODES OF MECHANICAL VENTILATION

21. Define the phrase "mode of ventilation" in your own words.

22. List the 10 maxims for understanding modes as described in this chapter.

   1. _____
   2. _____
   3. _____
   4. _____
   5. _____
   6. _____
   7. _____
   8. _____
   9. _____
  10. _____

23. What is inspiratory time? What does it equal?

24. What is expiratory time?

25. Define "work" as it relates to a patient's "work" of breathing.

26. How is a pressure support breath cycled?

27. Define patient triggering.

28. Define machine triggering.

29. Define patient cycling.

30. Define machine cycling.

31. List the three basic breath sequences and briefly describe each.

   A. _____
   B. _____
   C. _____

32. What is a target?

33. List the seven different targeting schemes used on commercially available ventilators.

A. _____

B. _____

C. _____

D. _____

E. _____

F. _____

G. _____

34. What are the three steps to classify a mode?

A. _____

B. _____

C. _____

TYPES OF VENTILATORS

35. Describe the volume and breath rate for conventional ventilation.

36. Describe some of the key features of the critical care ventilator.

37. Give four clinical reasons to use the noninvasive ventilator.

A. _____

B. _____

C. _____

D. _____

A 21-year-old patient is placed on a ventilator following a closed head injury. The physician desires to control this patient's ventilation to achieve a specific CO_2 level in the arterial blood.

38. Would you select volume or pressure ventilation to best achieve this goal?

39. Would you recommend a convention ICU ventilator or high-frequency option?

WHAT DOES THE NBRC SAY?

Circle the best answer.

40. A resident asks you to identify which of the basic modes of ventilation on an ICU ventilator will permit spontaneous breathing for a patient with neuromuscular disease. Which of the following would you select?
    1. CMV
    2. IMV
    3. CSV
       A. 1 and 3 only
       B. 1 and 2 only
       C. 2 and 3 only
       D. 1, 2, and 3

41. A patient in the early stages of ARDS is intubated. The physician states that he wishes to minimize the possibility of volutrauma or barotrauma. Which of the following modes would you recommend?
    A. Volume-controlled ventilation
    B. Manual ventilation
    C. CPAP
    D. Pressure-controlled ventilation

42. An 80-kg (176-lb) patient is being ventilated in volume control mode. During a ventilator check, the therapist notes that the compliance has decreased from 40 ml/cm H_2O to 35 ml/cm H_2O. What effect will this change in compliance have on volume?
    A. No effect
    B. Increased minute volume
    C. Decreased minute volume
    D. Decreased tidal volume

FOOD FOR THOUGHT

What types of ventilators are your hospitals using? Does practice vary between community hospitals and trauma centers? Find out what ventilator your clinical site is using and become familiar with it prior to attending that site. A good starting point for the new therapist is to learn a lot about the modes that are most commonly used in current practice where you live and where you do your clinical training. The best RTs can make the best of whatever mode is used in their institution while acting as resources for the nurses and physicians. They pull the other modes out of their bag of tricks when the opportunity arises, *but only after making themselves experts*. Introducing a new ventilator or new mode of ventilation is fraught with hazards if inservice training doesn't come along with the change.

46 Physiology of Ventilatory Support

WORD WIZARD

Look up the definitions in your glossary and write them out next to the words listed below.

1. Barotrauma _____

2. Time constant _____

3. Biotrauma _____

4. Transrespiratory pressure _____

5. Patient–ventilator asynchrony _____

6. Atelectrauma _____

7. Mean airway pressure _____

8. Transpulmonary pressure _____

PRESSURE AND PRESSURE GRADIENTS

9. Which pressure is responsible for maintaining normal alveolar inflation?

10. Which pressure gradient is required to expand the lungs and chest wall together?

11. Which pressure causes airflow in the airways?

12. What happens to transpulmonary pressure during normal inspiration? Exhalation?

   A. Inspiration _____

   B. Exhalation _____

13. What happens to transpulmonary pressure during inspiration with a negative-pressure ventilator? During exhalation?

   A. Inspiration _____

   B. Exhalation _____

14. What is "tank shock"?

15. What happens to the airway and pleural pressures during inspiration with a positive pressure ventilator?

EFFECTS OF MECHANICAL VENTILATION

Ventilation

16. A. What is the normal range of tidal volume during spontaneous breathing?
    B. What is the accepted tidal volume range for mechanical ventilation?

    A. _____ B. _____

17. Besides increasing the volume, how can you increase minute ventilation with the ventilator?

18. What effect does increasing the minute ventilation have on $PaCO_2$?

19. During spontaneous ventilation, where is gas mainly distributed? What about in positive pressure ventilation?

    A. Spontaneous _____

    B. PPV _____

20. How does perfusion, or blood flow, in the lung change during PPV?

Acid-Base Balance

21. Explain the importance of each the following as it relates to respiratory acidemia in a mechanically ventilated patient.

    A. Look at the patient _____

    B. Draw arterial blood _____

    C. Check electrolytes _____

    D. Check ECG _____

22. Explain the importance of each the following as it relates to respiratory alkalemia in a mechanically ventilated patient.

    A. Look at the patient _____

    B. Draw arterial blood _____

    C. Check electrolytes _____

    D. Check ECG _____

23. Explain the importance of each the following as it relates to metabolic acidemia and metabolic alkalemia in a mechanically ventilated patient.

Metabolic acidemia

A. Look at the patient _____

B. Draw arterial blood _____

Metabolic alkalemia

A. Look at the patient _____

B. Draw arterial blood _____

Oxygenation

24. Explain how mechanical ventilation improves oxygenation for each of the following causes of hypoxemia:

A. Hypoventilation _____

B. $\dot{V}/\dot{Q}$ mismatch _____

C. Shunt _____

25. What range of F_IO_2 can a modern ICU ventilator deliver?

26. State the formula for each of the following:

A. DO_2 _____

B. Alveolar air _____

C. Arterial oxygen content _____

D. Minute ventilation _____

LUNG MECHANICS

27. How long does it take for 95% of the alveoli in a normal lung to fill with air?

A. Time constants _____

B. Real time _____

What about 98% of alveoli? _____ 99%? _____

28. What are the two major factors that affect alveolar time constants?

A. _____

B. _____

29. You could help prolong the inspiratory phase for your patient with severe asthma by making the following adjustments:

A. Inspiratory time setting should be between _____ seconds.

B. What is the primary limiting factor in the airway? _____

C. How could you resolve this limitation? _____

331

30. You could help prolong the expiratory phase for your COPD patient by making the following adjustments:

A. Inspiratory times should between _____ seconds.

B. A common problem in these patients is _____ because of long time constants.

C. Respiratory rates are typically _____.

31. What is meant by the term "peak inspiratory pressure"? What's the abbreviation?

32. What is meant by the term "plateau pressure"? What's the symbol?

33. We can protect patient lungs from damage caused by pressure by maintaining plateau pressures at less than

_____ cm H$_2$O.

34. See if you know how to adjust mean airway pressure. Circle "T" for "true" if the choice is one that would *raise the mean airway pressure*. Circle "F" for false if it would not.

A. Increase peak pressure	T	F
B. Decrease inspiratory time	T	F
C. Synchronized IMV	T	F
D. Increase PEEP levels	T	F
E. Constant pressure pattern (PC mode, decelerating ramp flow)	T	F

35. How does increasing airway pressure affect the FRC and oxygenation?

A. FRC _____

B. Oxygenation _____

36. What will happen to compliance when too much PEEP is applied? Could you adjust the PEEP based on the

changes in compliance? _____

37. The pressure-volume curve is useful for establishing relationship of the lung-thorax in patients with ARDS. Name each of the following:

A. Lower inflection point: _____ or _____

B. Upper inflection point: _____

38. Why does dead space increase during mechanical ventilation?

WORK OF BREATHING

39. Work of breathing (WOB) consists of what two components?

A. _____

B. _____

40. Measuring WOB at the bedside is difficult. What is normal WOB? What three variables does the experienced therapist use to determine whether WOB is excessive?

Normal WOB: _____

    A. _____

    B. _____

    C. _____

PULMONARY EFFECTS OF POSITIVE PRESSURE MECHANICAL VENTILATION

41. List two negative pulmonary effects of too much PEEP.

    A. _____

    B. _____

42. Why can PEEP be a problem with severe unilateral lung disease?

43. Compare square flow patterns with descending ramp.

PHYSIOLOGIC EFFECTS OF VENTILATORY MODES

44. Identify two potential harmful effects of inappropriate trigger-level setting when a patient's ventilation is in CMV mode.

    A. _____

    B. _____

45. When is VC-CMV indicated?

46. When would you choose PC-CMV over VC-CMV?

47. What are the possible benefits of APRV?

48. When is PSV useful?

49. Bilevel PAP was originally developed for treatment of obstructive sleep apnea. It has also been shown to be useful in acute care settings with COPD exacerbations. Explain.

50. How does proportional-assist ventilation (PAV) work?

51. Compare PAV to neutrally adjusted ventilatory assist (NAVA).

52. Automatic tube compensation is not a mode of ventilation. What is it really? What does the RT input?

53. How is patient-ventilator interaction monitored in adaptive control/dual control mode?

Patient Positioning to Optimize Oxygenation and Ventilation

54. What group of patients is most likely to benefit from prone positioning?

55. What should be monitored when changing positioning of patients?

CARDIOVASCULAR EFFECTS OF POSITIVE PRESSURE MECHANICAL VENTILATION

56. Briefly explain the negative effects of PPV on the heart. What are these effects dependent on?

57. How can you use the ventilator to temporarily manage increased ICP?

58. Explain the mechanism behind the drop in urine output in ventilated patients.

   A. Direct _____

   B. Indirect _____

59. Why is sedation necessary for the management of a patient in the ICU?

60. When using a chest cuirass and poncho-type negative-pressure ventilators, what problems can result in hypoventilation?

    A. _____

    B. _____

61. Positive pressure ventilation has long been associated with barotrauma. List three of the clinical signs of pneumothorax.

    A. Chest motion _____

    B. Percussion note _____

    C. Breath sounds _____

62. Tension pneumothorax is life threatening in a ventilated patient. How and where is this treated?

    A. How?

    B. Where in the chest?

63. What is volutrauma, and how is it prevented?

64. Oxygen toxicity may damage lung tissue. Every effort should be made to reduce the F_IO_2 to what value?

65. List three ways to reduce the risk of ventilator-associated pneumonias.

    A. Positioning _____

    B. Endotracheal tubes _____

    C. Reduce condensates _____

Fill in the blanks.

66. Positive physiologic effects of PPV include improved _____ and ventilation, and decreased _____ of breathing.

67. Research indicates better ventilator synchrony and gas exchange with the _____ flow pattern than the _____ flow pattern.

68. _____-triggering appears to be a better choice than _____-triggering when it is available on the ventilator.

69. PEEP is applied to restore _____ in restrictive disease and _____ the airways in obstructive disease.

70. Positive pressure ventilation is detrimental to the $\dot{V}/\dot{Q}$ ratio primarily by shifting to areas that are less _____.

71. PPV may cause hepatic and gastrointestinal malfunction primarily due to decreased _____ of capillary tissue beds.

CASE STUDY

Part 1

A trauma patient is stabilized after a motor vehicle accident. He is intubated and transported to the ICU, where you place him on a ventilator. As soon as you put him on the machine, his blood pressure falls dramatically.

72. What should you do (right away!)?

73. What is the most likely cause of hypotension in a trauma patient who has been placed on positive pressure ventilation?

Part 2

Two days later, the patient has developed poor lung compliance and hypoxemia associated with noncardiogenic pulmonary edema (ARDS). He is being ventilated on VC-CMV, frequency of 12, tidal volume of 700 mL, +15 cm H_2O PEEP, and F_IO_2 0.70. Blood gases show pH 7.37, $PaCO_2$ 38, and PaO_2 55. Peak inspiratory pressure is 60 cm H_2O, and plateau pressure is 50 cm H_2O.

74. There are two serious problems here. Identify them.

   A. Serious problem No. 1 _____

   B. Serious problem No. 2 _____

75. What change(s) in ventilator strategy would you suggest?

   A. Problem No. 1

   B. Problem No. 2

WHAT DOES THE NBRC SAY?

Review each of the common modes of ventilation.

FOOD FOR THOUGHT

76. If the newest modes of ventilation are not proven to alter patient outcomes, why should we use them?

77. Patients on ventilators have a really high incidence of GI bleeding. Why is GI bleeding such a big deal to RTs?

47 Patient Ventilator Interaction

WORD WIZARD

State the cause for each of the following terms and how you would correct the problem.

1. Missed triggering

   A. Cause: _____

   B. Modification to correct: _____

2. Double triggering

   A. Cause: _____

   B. Modification to correct: _____

3. Auto-triggering

   A. Cause: _____

   B. Modification to correct: _____

4. Reverse triggering

   A. Cause: _____

   B. Modification to correct: _____

5. Delayed triggering

   A. Cause: _____

   B. Modification to correct: _____

6. Mode asynchrony

   A. Cause: _____

   B. Modification to correct: _____

7. Cycle asynchrony

   A. Cause: _____

   B. Modification to correct: _____

EFFECT OF POOR PATIENT-VENTILATOR INTERACTION ON OUTCOME

8. What is patient-ventilator interaction, and why is it critical during mechanical ventilation?

9. How can poor patient-ventilator interactions negatively affect the patient?

10. List four issues with an artificial airway that can cause poor patient-ventilator.

    A. _____

    B. _____

    C. _____

    D. _____

11. List three problems that can cause rapid deterioration in the patient's clinical status.

    A. _____

    B. _____

    C. _____

VARIABLES CONTROLLED DURING MECHANICAL VENTILATION

12. Why are the modes proportional assist ventilation (PAV) and neutrally adjusted ventilatory assist (NAVA) least likely to cause asynchrony?

13. In PAV and NAVA, what happens when patient effort increases?

TYPES OF ASYNCHRONY

14. When does flow asynchrony occur? Is there a mode it is more likely to occur in?

15. What must you do to prevent flow asynchrony?

16. In which two modes of ventilation is mode asynchrony least likely to occur?

    A. _____

    B. _____

17. In which mode of mechanical ventilation is cycle asynchrony most likely to occur? Why?

FOOD FOR THOUGHT

Mechanical ventilation is not a cookie-cutter modality. There is no one mode or one setting that will ensure the most appropriate patient-ventilator interaction occurs. The only thing that makes a difference is how the RT manages the patient!

48 Initiating and Adjusting Invasive Ventilatory Support

Let's go right to the cases and find out if you understand how to initiate and adjust ventilatory support. This chapter will use case studies to help you understand how to initiate and adjust invasive ventilatory support. Five basic types of lungs and 10 specific disorders can account for almost every case of mechanical ventilation. Table 48-4 covers most of the bases and can help you tremendously.

Case 1

A 5-foot 5-inch, 60-kg (132-lb) young woman attempted suicide by drug overdose. She is unconscious and breathing slowly and shallowly. The emergency physician elects to intubate this patient.

1. What size ET tube would be appropriate for an adult female?
   A. 6.0-mm inside diameter
   B. 7.0-mm outside diameter
   C. 7.5-mm inside diameter
   D. 8.0-mm inside diameter

2. In the emergency setting, how will you assess proper tube placement?
   1. Auscultate the chest.
   2. Auscultate the epigastrium.
   3. Attach an exhaled O_2 monitor.
   4. Observe chest wall motion.
      A. 1 and 2 only
      B. 1 and 3 only
      C. 2, 3, and 4 only
      D. 1, 2, and 4 only

After the intubation is completed, a small amount of white secretions are suctioned from the airway. The physician requests a room air ABG at this point. Results show:

pH	7.25
$PaCO_2$	60 mm Hg
PaO_2	55 mm Hg
HCO_3^-	26 mEq/L

Vital signs are:

HR	115
BP	125/75
RR	26
Temp	37

A chest film is taken, which reveals the tip of the endotracheal tube to be 4 cm above the carina with no sign of a pneumothorax.

3. What action would you recommend in regard to the ET tube placement?
   A. Advance the tube 2 to 3 cm.
   B. Withdraw the tube 2 to 3 cm.
   C. Maintain current placement.
   D. Remove the tube and insert a laryngeal mask airway.

4. The ABG results are interpreted as _____.
   A. metabolic acidosis with severe hypoxemia
   B. respiratory acidosis with moderate hypoxemia
   C. partially compensated respiratory alkalosis with mild hypoxemia
   D. partially compensated metabolic alkalosis with moderate hypoxemia

The patient is transported to the ICU. The physician requests that you initiate mechanical ventilation.

5. Calculate ideal body weight.
   A. 45 kg
   B. 59 kg
   C. 65 kg
   D. 130 kg

6. Which of the following volumes would you recommend?
   A. 410 ml
   B. 610 ml
   C. 710 ml
   D. 810 ml

7. What mode and rate would you select?
   A. PSV, 10 cm H_2O
   B. VC-IMV, 6
   C. VC-CMV, 12
   D. VC-CMV, 22

8. What type of humidification system would you recommend for this patient?
   A. Heated wick humidifier set at 35° C
   B. HME
   C. Heated passover humidifier
   D. Bubble humidifier

Three days later, the patient is alert and weaning is initiated. When the rate is decreased to 5, however, the patient's spontaneous respiratory rate rises to 30 and tidal volumes drop to 200 ml.

9. To help resolve this problem you might recommend initiation of _____.
   A. CMV
   B. AC
   C. PSV
   D. APRV

Paramedics bring a 5-foot 2-inch, 50-kg (110-lb) 65-year-old woman with a history of COPD to the emergency department for treatment of dyspnea. She is wearing a nasal cannula set at 2 L/min. ABGs are drawn. Results show:

pH	7.30
$PaCO_2$	70 mm Hg
PaO_2	45 mm Hg
HCO_3^-	34 mEq/L

Vital signs are:

HR	100
BP	100/70
RR	34
Temp	39

Noninvasive positive pressure breathing is attempted with bilevel ventilation, but the patient is unable to tolerate the mask and fights the system. A decision is made to intubate and initiate mechanical ventilation. The patient is given a small amount of sedation and intubated nasally with a 6.5-mm ID tube. Settings are:

Mode	VC-IMV
Rate	14
V_T	400 ml
F_IO_2	0.28
PEEP	0
Peak flow	20 LPM
Flow pattern	Decelerating ramp
Sensitivity	1.5 cm H_2O below baseline

10. How long should you wait before drawing an ABG to assess the results of these settings?
    A. 5 minutes
    B. 20 minutes
    C. 40 minutes
    D. 60 minutes

11. What is the maximum desirable plateau pressure during mechanical ventilation?
    A. 15 cm H_2O
    B. 25 cm H_2O
    C. 28 cm H_2O
    D. 40 cm H_2O

During your first patient-ventilator system assessment, the following observations are made.

PIP	40 cm H_2O
Plateau	35 cm H_2O
Set rate	14
Total rate	25
Exhaled V_T	425 ml
I:E ratio	1:1.5

12. What high-pressure alarm limit should you set?
    A. 35 cm H_2O
    B. 45 cm H_2O
    C. 50 cm H_2O
    D. 65 cm H_2O

13. What value should you set for the low-minute ventilation alarm?
    A. 2.0 L
    B. 3.0 L
    C. 4.0 L
    D. 5.0 L

14. Which of the following would result in a lower work of breathing for this patient?
    1. Addition of 100 ml mechanical dead space
    2. Initiation of PSV at 5 cm H_2O
    3. Changing to flow-triggering 2 L/min
    4. Addition of 10 cm H_2O PEEP
        A. 1 and 2 only
        B. 2 and 3 only
        C. 1 and 3 only
        D. 2, 3, and 4 only

15. What action should you take to increase the I:E ratio?
    A. Increase the peak flow.
    B. Increase the tidal volume.
    C. Increase the set rate.
    D. Increase the F_IO_2.

16. What I:E ratio would provide sufficient time for exhalation and prevent auto-PEEP in this COPD patient?
    A. 1:1
    B. 1:2
    C. 1:4
    D. 1:10

Case 3

A 5-foot 6-inch woman who weighs 100 kg (220 lb) is in the ICU following surgery for multiple injuries sustained in a motor vehicle accident. She has an arterial line and a pulmonary artery catheter in place. Her chest radiograph shows bilateral infiltrates consistent with ARDS. The ET tube is in good position.

Current ventilator settings are:

Mode	VC- CMV
V_T	800
Rate	12
F_IO_2	0.70
PEEP	5 cm H_2O
Peak flow	60 L/min, decelerating ramp
Sensitivity	1.0 cm H_2O below baseline

17. What is this patient's approximate ideal body weight?
    A. 50 kg
    B. 60 kg
    C. 80 kg
    D. 100 kg

18. What initial tidal volume would you recommend to prevent further lung injury?
    A. 460 ml
    B. 660 ml
    C. 720 ml
    D. Maintain current setting

The following data are obtained:

HR	110, NSR with occasional PVCs
BP	110/75 mm Hg
SpO_2	88%
PA	38/8 mm Hg
PCWP	12 mm Hg
CO	5.8 L/min
SvO_2	59%

19. With regard to the patient's oxygenation, what action would you recommend?
    A. Increase the F_IO_2.
    B. Increase the PEEP.
    C. Add mechanical dead space.
    D. Maintain current settings.

A PEEP trial is conducted with the following results.

PEEP	Cstat	PaO_2	CO
5	22	57	5.8
10	25	66	5.7
15	30	72	5.9
20	25	77	5.2
25	22	85	4.8

20. What PEEP level would you recommend?
    A. 5
    B. 10
    C. 15
    D. 20
    E. 25

The patient continues to deteriorate over the next 2 days. Her compliance and PaO_2 have decreased, while PIP has increased to 60 cm H_2O to maintain a normal $PaCO_2$.

21. Which of the following ventilator modes could be considered as alternatives?
    1. PC-CMV
    2. VC-IMV
    3. APRV
    4. CPAP
        A. 1 and 3 only
        B. 2 and 3 only
        C. 2 and 4 only
        D. 1 and 4 only

22. Which of these techniques are used with ARDS with a P/F ratio less than 100 to reduce lung injury or improve oxygenation?
    1. Expiratory retard
    2. Prone positioning
    3. Permissive hypercapnia
    4. Unilateral lung ventilation
        A. 1 and 2 only
        B. 2 and 3 only
        C. 1 and 4 only
        D. 3 and 4 only

A respiratory student who fell down the stairs while reading *Egan's* suffered a closed-head injury. The student is 5 feet 5 inches tall and weighs 60 kg. ICP and blood pressure are elevated. She is being ventilated with these settings.

Mode	VC-CMV
Rate	10
V_T	600
F_IO_2	0.30
PEEP	0

Blood gases on these settings are:

pH	7.40
$PaCO_2$	40
PaO_2	55
HCO_3^-	24

23. This blood gas should be interpreted as _____.
    A. normal with moderate hypoxemia
    B. respiratory alkalosis with mild hypoxemia
    C. compensated respiratory acidosis with severe hypoxemia
    D. compensated metabolic alkalosis with moderate hypoxemia

24. With regard to the oxygenation, what change would you suggest?
    A. Increase the PEEP.
    B. Increase the rate.
    C. Change to APRV.
    D. Increase the F_IO_2.

25. With regard to the ventilation, what change would you suggest?
    A. Increase the rate.
    B. Increase the tidal volume.
    C. Change to IMV.
    D. Add mechanical dead space.

26. What is the formula for calculating the rate needed to produce a desired change in $PaCO_2$?
    A. $PaCO_2$ measured $\times$ set rate $\div$ $PaCO_2$ desired
    B. $PaCO_2$ desired $\times$ set rate $\div$ $PaCO_2$ measured
    C. $PaCO_2$ measured $\times$ $PaCO_2$ desired $\div$ set rate
    D. $PaCO_2$ measured $\times$ PaO_2 measured $\div$ set rate

27. What rate would you suggest for this patient if the desired $PaCO_2$ is 30 mm Hg?
    A. 8
    B. 10
    C. 14
    D. 18

28. How long should you maintain a head injury patient in a hyperventilated state?
    A. 2 to 4 hours
    B. 6 to 8 hours
    C. 12 to 24 hours
    D. 24 to 48 hours

A 5-foot 7-inch, 27-year-old woman who weighs 140 lb with a long history of asthma including previous intubation and mechanical ventilation presents in the emergency department with high-pitched, diffuse wheezing. She is barely able to talk because of her dyspnea. She has not responded to two consecutive SVN treatments with 5 mg of albuterol and 0.5 mg of Atrovent. Peak flows are not measurable, and SpO_2 is 92% on 2 L via nasal cannula. She is using her accessory muscles to breathe and has some intercostal retractions on inspiration. She is started on IV Solu-Medrol, continuous bronchodilator therapy, and ECG monitoring. One hour later, she is lethargic and breath sounds are virtually absent. You draw an ABG with the following results:

pH	7.29
$PaCO_2$	55 mm Hg
PaO_2	64 mm Hg
HCO_3^-	24 mmol
SaO_2	90%

29. What action would you recommend at this time?
   A. Continuation of present therapy
   B. Oral intubation with 7.5 ET tube and mechanical ventilation
   C. Trial of NIV via bilevel mask ventilation
   D. Tracheostomy and mechanical ventilation

30. The emergency physician elects to move the patient to the MICU as soon as she is stabilized. You assist in the transport. In the ICU, you are asked to set up the ventilator. Which of the following would you select?
   A. VC-IMV 14, 400, 0.40 F_IO_2, +3 PEEP, +5 PSV
   B. VC-CMV 12, 350, +5 PEEP, 0.40 F_IO_2
   C. APRV high PEEP 30, low PEEP 0, 0.60 F_IO_2, 1-second release time
   D. PSV 10 cm H_2O, 0.30 F_IO_2

31. What pharmacologic agent is recommended at this time?
   A. Inhaled corticosteroids
   B. Sedation with midazolam
   C. Paralysis with cisatracurium besylate
   D. Respiratory stimulus with doxapram

32. Which of the following are major concerns when ventilating severe asthmatics?
   1. Pulmonary barotrauma
   2. Development of auto-PEEP
   3. Ventilator asynchrony
   4. High airway pressures
      A. 1 and 2 only
      B. 1, 3, and 4 only
      C. 2, 3, and 4 only
      D. 1, 2, 3, and 4 only

33. An appropriate peak flow and flow pattern for this patient would include
   A. 40 L/min with a decelerating flow waveform.
   B. 20 L/min with a square flow waveform.
   C. 100 L/min with a sine wave flow pattern.
   D. 50 L/min with an accelerating flow waveform.

34. What alteration to the mode of ventilation might be useful to prevent barotrauma and improve comfort?
    A. Addition of mechanical dead space
    B. Using a heated humidifier
    C. Switching to pressure control
    D. Utilizing inverse ratio ventilation

Case 6

A 6-foot, 176-lb 66-year-old man has been brought to the SICU following coronary artery bypass graft surgery. He has no history of lung disease. He is intubated with a No. 8 oral ET tube. The anesthesiologist asks you to select ventilator settings.

35. What tidal volume is appropriate for this postoperative patient?
    A. 550 ml
    B. 660 ml
    C. 800 ml
    D. 950 ml

36. Why should you add PEEP to the system?
    A. To prevent auto-PEEP
    B. To prevent atelectasis
    C. To prevent cardiogenic pulmonary edema
    D. To prevent barotrauma

37. What is your primary goal for this patient?
    A. Prevent ventilator-associated barotrauma.
    B. Prevent ventilator-associated pneumonia.
    C. Control air trapping.
    D. Wean and extubate as quickly as possible.

WHAT DOES THE NBRC SAY?

Circle the best answer.

38. A patient with CHF is placed on the ventilator with proper tube placement confirmed. The respiratory therapist should
    A. obtain a sputum sample for culture.
    B. assess changes in intracranial pressure.
    C. assess changes in blood pressure.
    D. obtain a chest x-ray.

39. A patient is receiving mechanical ventilation via VC-CMV with a mandatory rate of 14. Peak inspiratory pressures are in the low 50s. The physician wants to maintain the mean airway pressure but lower the peak pressure. What would you recommend?
    A. Increase the mandatory rate.
    B. Increase the inspiratory flow.
    C. Initiate pressure-controlled ventilation.
    D. Initiate IMV with pressure support.

40. What is an appropriate range for respiratory rate (f) when using high-frequency oscillation ventilation in adults?
    A. 1-2 Hz
    B. 3-5 Hz
    C. 10-15 Hz
    D. 20-30 Hz

41. A patient with ARDS due to trauma from a motor vehicle crash is placed on mechanical ventilation. The man is 182 cm (6 feet) tall and weighs 100 kg (220 lb). With respect to ventilator settings, what tidal volume would you recommend?
    A. 460 ml
    B. 560 ml
    C. 660 ml
    D. 800 ml

42. An apneic patient is placed on mechanical ventilation following surgery. What range of rates is typical for initiating mechanical ventilation on an adult patient?
    A. 4-8
    B. 8-12
    C. 12-16
    D. 16-20

43. A patient is being mechanically ventilated in CMV mode. When the patient begins to inhale, airway pressure drops to –4 cm H_2O below baseline before a breath is started. What control needs to be adjusted?
    A. Frequency
    B. PEEP
    C. Pressure support
    D. Sensitivity

44. A patient with ARDS is being mechanically ventilated with a PEEP of 10 cm H_2O and an F_IO_2 of 0.80. When the patient is removed from the ventilator for suctioning, he experiences decreased oxygen saturation and increased heart rate. What should the respiratory therapist recommend?
    A. Decreasing the PEEP to 5 cm H_2O
    B. Changing to a closed suction system
    C. Giving SVN with albuterol 2.5 mg
    D. Increasing the F_IO_2 on the ventilator

45. A 70-kg patient is ventilated on VC-IMV mode with a rate of 8, tidal volume of 700, F_IO_2 of 0.40, PEEP of 4 cm H_2O, pressure support of 4 cm H_2O, and inspiratory flow rate of 45 L/min. The patient is breathing 22 times per minute in between the machine breaths with a tidal volume of 150 ml. What change should the respiratory therapist recommend?
    A. Increasing the peak inspiratory flow rate
    B. Increasing the respiratory rate
    C. Increasing the set tidal volume
    D. Increasing the pressure support

46. A 50-kg adult female is mechanically ventilated following a cardiac arrest. What tidal volume setting is recommended for this patient?
    A. 250 ml
    B. 350 ml
    C. 450 ml
    D. 550 ml

FOOD FOR THOUGHT

47. What are the common ventilator modes where you are training or working? Practice them in the lab.

49 Noninvasive Ventilation

WORD WIZARD

We've been looking for less invasive ways to help people breathe since the first invasive airway management with tracheostomy tubes was performed 350 years ago. In the 1930s a rubber inflatable device called a _____ was strapped to the abdomen to help patients with _____ disease to help move the diaphragm. Later, a _____ bed was designed to help with weaning. Motion _____ was a hazard of the bed. Negative pressure ventilators like the _____ lung were used to treat polio patients but were large and bulky. A chest _____ covers only the chest and looks like a turtle shell.

INDICATIONS FOR NONINVASIVE VENTILATION

1. What is the primary goal of noninvasive ventilation (NIV)?

2. List three potential benefits of NIV in the acute care setting.

    A. _____

    B. _____

    C. _____

3. In the acute care setting, NIV is indicated for numerous conditions. List at least four.

    A. _____

    B. _____

    C. _____

    D. _____

4. NIV is also indicated for the long-term care setting. List four conditions.

    A. _____

    B. _____

    C. _____

    D. _____

5. How is the need for ventilatory assistance established?

   A. Respiratory rate _____

   B. Dyspnea _____

   C. $PaCO_2$ and pH _____

   D. P/F ratio _____

6. List at least four exclusion criteria for NIV.

   A. _____

   B. _____

   C. _____

   D. _____

7. What is the standard of care for acute COPD exacerbation or cardiogenic pulmonary edema in the acute care setting?

8. Compare CPAP to bilevel noninvasive ventilation in the treatment of acute cardiogenic pulmonary edema. When does bilevel outperform CPAP?

9. Describe the two basic parts of the decision-making process for a patient with chronic restrictive thoracic disease.

   A.

   B.

EQUIPMENT USED FOR NONINVASIVE VENTILATION

10. What is an interface?

11. Which type of patient interface is most commonly used for NIV? Which is usually the best choice for treating patients in acute respiratory failure?

12. What is the key factor in patient tolerance and NIV efficacy?

13. Compare nasal mask sizing and oronasal mask sizing techniques. Which is more susceptible to leaks?

14. List three disadvantages associated with oronasal masks.

   A. _____

   B. _____

   C. _____

15. Patients with what complication would benefit from a total face mask?

TYPES OF MECHANICAL VENTILATORS AND MODES OF VENTILATION

16. Define the following terms:

   A. CPAP: _____

   B. IPAP: _____

   C. EPAP: _____

17. What happens to tidal volume when you increase the EPAP without increasing the IPAP?

18. What are some of the problems with using critical care ventilators to deliver mask ventilation? What may help?

19. How can you recognize active exhalation on the ventilator's graphics?

20. What are two ways to correct the problem of active exhalation?

   A. _____

   B. _____

21. List two advantageous performance characteristics of home care ventilators.

   A. _____

   B. _____

22. What is the temperature for heated humidity when using NIV? Why is it used?

23. How should your patient be positioned when applying NIV?

24. How should you prepare the patient for the experience?

25. What pressure could open the esophagus?

26. What tidal volumes are you aiming for when applying NIV? Which control do you adjust if the volume is too low?

    A. Goal: _____

    B. Adjust: _____

27. Which two adjustments can be made to improve oxygenation?

28. Fill in the chart below regarding possible side effects and complications of NIV.

	Possible Solutions
Interface-Related Side Effects	
Discomfort	
Erythema	
Claustrophobia	
Pressure ulcer	
Skin rash	
Air–Pressure-Related or Flow-Related Side Effects	
Nasal congestion	
Nasal dryness	
Sinus or ear pain	
Eye irritation	
Gastric distention	
Serious Complications	
Aspiration	
Pneumothorax	
Hypotension	

Mary Mac is a 61-year-old female with a 60-pack-year history of smoking who was diagnosed with COPD 7 years ago. She is currently being treated on the general floor for community-acquired pneumonia. She has been intubated twice because of exacerbation of COPD and is currently complaining of dyspnea. Vital signs are heart rate 96 beats/min, blood pressure 138/86 mm Hg, respiratory rate 22 breaths/min, and SpO_2 90% on a nasal cannula at 6 L/min. ABGs reveal pH 7.25, $PaCO_2$ 66 mm Hg, and, PaO_2 59 mm Hg. She is very anxious and tripoding.

29. What treatment would you initiate at this time?

30. What is your goal with your care of Mary Mac?

31. Where would you initiate the treatment you choose?

Mary is now stable and is requiring Atrovent.

32. Can this be given if she is currently receiving NIV? If yes, where would you position the nebulizer? Where would you position an MDI?

33. Mary has been on NIV for 3 hours, and she is not improving. What treatment would you suggest to the physician?

WHAT DOES THE NBRC SAY?

Questions 34-37 refer to the following scenario. Circle the best answer.

A 60-kg, 70-year-old patient with COPD does not wish to be intubated and has an advance directive supporting his wishes. The patient is admitted to the medical ICU in respiratory failure. ABGs reveal pH 7.25, $PaCO_2$ 66 mm Hg, and PaO_2 50 mm Hg.

34. What mode of therapy would the respiratory therapist recommend in this situation?
    A. Nasal cannula at 6 L/min
    B. Nonrebreathing mask at 10 L/min
    C. Continuous positive airway pressure (CPAP)
    D. Noninvasive ventilation (NIV)

35. NIV is initiated on spontaneous mode with F_iO_2 0.40, IPAP of 8 cm H_2O, and EPAP of 2 cm H_2O. ABGs reveal pH 7.29, $PaCO_2$ 54, PaO_2 52, and HCO_3 30. The respiratory therapist should recommend what change in regard to the carbon dioxide levels?
    A. Increase the respiratory rate setting.
    B. Increase the tidal volume setting.
    C. Increase the IPAP.
    D. Increase the EPAP.

36. What should the RT recommend to improve oxygenation?
    A. Increase the respiratory rate setting.
    B. Increase the tidal volume setting.
    C. Increase the IPAP.
    D. Increase the EPAP.

37. What exhaled tidal volume would you target for this patient?
    A. 200 ml
    B. 350 ml
    C. 475 ml
    D. 600 ml

FOOD FOR THOUGHT

As an RT you should always be your patient's advocate. The last thing you should want to do is intubate and mechanically ventilate a patient. If you have to, you should always be thinking of how to get patients off the ventilator and breathing on their own again. Your knowledge and understanding of NIV and cardiopulmonary pathophysiology can help. So, study, read, and learn! Your patients are depending on it.

50 Extracorporeal Life Support (ECLS)

WORD WIZARD

Match the following terms with their definitions as they relate to extracorporeal life support.

_____ Venous reservoir

_____ Sweep flow

_____ VA ECMO

_____ Pump flow

_____ VV ECMO

_____ AV ECMO

_____ Activated clotting time

A. The primary test for anticoagulation at the bedside.
B. Primarily for CO_2 removal at low pump flows and requires the patient's own hemodynamics to pump blood through the oxygenator.
C. Support is partial cardiopulmonary bypass, providing both cardiac and pulmonary support.
D. The bladder.
E. Dependent on the patient's preload and afterload.
F. Gas flow.
G. Only provides pulmonary support.

EXTRACORPOREAL LIFE SUPPORT (ECLS)

1. What are the primary goals of extracorporeal membrane oxygenation (ECMO)?

2. What are the three general types of ECMO?

   A. _____

   B. _____

   C. _____

3. Describe the qualities that make an RT a prime candidate as an ECMO specialist.

4. What two ways is ECMO primarily used in the pediatric and adult patient?

   A. _____

   B. _____

5. Describe normal cardiopulmonary physiology during circulation of the blood beginning in the right heart.

6. What two components make up the total oxygen content in the blood?

   A. _____

   B. _____

7. ECMO equipment has what task?

8. Describe an ECMO circuit. Is short or long tubing best?

9. Why is tubing length particularly important in the newborn population?

10. When blood is drained from the patient, where does it go?

11. How is the ECMO system powered?

12. What three situations can cause excessive negative pressure on the right atrium?

    A. _____

    B. _____

    C. _____

13. When adjusting the blender, what are the saturation and PO_2 goals for the hemoglobin leaving the oxygenator?

14. Why does CO_2 diffuse into the sweep fibers?

15. How does sweep flow relate to CO_2 elimination?

16. What is a typical sweep flow to pump flow ratio?

17. What additional ECMO equipment is needed?

ANTICOAGULATION MANAGEMENT ON ECMO

18. What is the most common medication used as an anticoagulant during ECMO?

19. List three factors that can affect the activated clotting time (ACT) in ECMO patients.

    A. _____

    B. _____

    C. _____

20. What does the "M" number mean as it relates to cannulas?

21. What three characteristics are considered when sizing cannulas?

    A. _____

    B. _____

    C. _____

TYPES OF SUPPORT

22. Give a detailed explanation for each of the following types of ECMO.

    A. VV ECMO _____

    B. VA ECMO _____

    C. AV ECMO _____

23. How many cannulas need to be placed for VA ECMO? Where are they placed?

24. Give indications for each of the following types of ECMO.

    A. VV ECMO _____

    B. VA ECMO _____

    C. AV ECMO _____

25. Give a disadvantage of VA ECMO.

26. What advantages does VV ECMO have over VA ECMO?

27. List six physiologic complications of ECMO.

    A. _____

    B. _____

    C. _____

    D. _____

    E. _____

    F. _____

WEANING AND DECANNULATION FROM ECMO

28. Describe the weaning process for VA and VV ECMO. Include mechanical ventilator parameters.

    A. VA _____

    B. VV _____

SUMMARY CHECKLIST

29. What is a major advantage of ECMO as it relates to ventilatory support?

30. Why is anticoagulant therapy necessary during ECMO?

FOOD FOR THOUGHT

Even though ECMO is currently not on the NBRC matrix, study hard because it soon will be. An RT's role in patient care is becoming more and more advanced, so read the literature and get ready!

51 Monitoring the Patient in the Intensive Care Unit

The best monitor is a knowledgeable, observant, and dedicated health care professional.

Donald F. Egan, MD

WORD WIZARD

Match these key terms to the definitions that follow.

Terms	Definitions
1. _____ Afterload	A. Pressure the ventricle has to contract against.
	B. Pressure stretching the ventricle at the onset of contraction.
2. _____ Swan-Ganz catheter	C. Unreal events seen on monitors often caused by movement.
3. _____ Qs/Qt	D. Popular system for measuring neurologic impairment.
4. _____ Apache score	E. Hemodynamic monitoring device placed in the pulmonary artery.
	F. Amount of wasted ventilation per breath.
5. _____ VD/Vt	G. Techniques for lung mapping.
6. _____ EIT and ARM	H. Popular acute illness index.
7. _____ Preload	I. Bedside test for respiratory muscle strength.
8. _____ Maximal inspiratory pressure	J. Physiologic shunt.
9. _____ Glasgow Coma Scale score	
10. _____ Artifacts	

PRINCIPLES OF MONITORING

Monitoring Oxygenation

11. Describe the difference between noninvasive and invasive monitoring.

12. How are exchange of oxygen and the removal of carbon dioxide best monitored invasively? What noninvasive test can be used for immediate continuous assessment of oxygenation?

    A. Invasive: _____

    B. Noninvasive: _____

13. Tissue oxygenation depends on several factors. List four of them.

    A. _____

    B. _____

    C. _____

    D. _____

14. What are the most serious clinical limitations of using pulse oximetry to assess respiratory status?

15. What is tissue oxygen sensing?

16. What does the Fick equation measure?

17. How are the following measurements useful when monitoring an ICU patient?

A. PaO_2/F_IO_2 ratio: _____

B. $(P(A - a)O_2)$: _____

C. OI: _____

18. What does the Berlin definition of ARDS include?

A. _____

B. _____

C. _____

D. _____

E. _____

19. What is the most accurate way to measure oxygenation efficiency? What is the formula?

A. _____

B. _____

20. What four factors are included in the Murray lung injury score?

A. _____

B. _____

C. _____

D. _____

MONITORING VENTILATION

21. When is ventilation considered adequate?

22. Describe a patient in which capnometry would be a useful tool.

23. Measuring physiologic dead space assesses efficiency of ventilation. State the modified Bohr equation.

$V_D/V_T =$ _____

24. List the normal and critical values for dead space–to–tidal volume ratio.

A. Normal _____   _____

B. Critical is > _____ and predicts failure to wean.

MONITORING LUNG AND CHEST WALL MECHANICS

25. The pressure–volume curve is a ventilator graphic that can show compliance and lower inflection points. The lower inflection point may help you set what ventilator parameter?

26. The upper inflection point may point out what problem?

27. What is normal compliance? How is it calculated?

28. What is the formula for calculating airway resistance?

R_{aw} = _____

29. What is normal airway resistance? What's normal for a ventilated patient?

A. Normal _____

B. Ventilated patients _____

30. What is the safe maximum value for peak pressure? _____

31. What are the maximum safe plateau pressures? _____

32. Explain how adjustment of extrinsic PEEP is related to the level of intrinsic (auto) PEEP.

33. Define stress index. What can it be useful in determining?

34. What is the primary goal of manipulating MAP?

35. What is the simplest way to monitor a patient's work of breathing?

36. What is a $P_{0.1}$? What two factors influence this measurement?

37. What are the benefits of measuring MIP compared to VC?

A. _____

B. _____

MONITORING THE PATIENT–VENTILATOR SYSTEM

38. Briefly discuss the areas that are part of a patient-ventilator system check.

A. Airway _____

B. Vent settings _____

C. Gas exchange _____

D. Respiratory mechanics _____

E. The patient _____

F. Alarms _____

G. Other issues _____

39. How can ventilator graphics be used in the patient-ventilator system check?

A. _____

B. _____

C. _____

D. _____

E. _____

40. Explain the key steps listed below regarding a patient-ventilator system check.

A. Before entering the room

B. Explain

C. Observe

D. Drain

E. Airway

F. Inspect

G. Auscultate

H. Note pressures (at least three)

I. Graphics

CARDIAC AND CARDIOVASCULAR MONITORING

41. What is the most common noninvasive tool used to monitor the conduction system of the heart?

42. Identify the two main sites for arterial cannulation in adults.

    A. _____

    B. _____

43. What are the two indications for an indwelling arterial line?

    A. _____

    B. _____

44. List six conditions that suggest insertion of a pulmonary artery catheter.

    A. _____

    B. _____

    C. _____

    D. _____

    E. _____

    F. _____

45. List the normal values for these parameters.

    A. Central venous pressure (CVP) _____

    B. Right atrial pressure (RA) _____

    C. Pulmonary _____

        1. Systolic _____

        2. Diastolic _____

    D. Pulmonary artery wedge pressure (PWP, PCWP, PAWP) _____

    E. Cardiac output (CO) _____

    F. Cardiac index (CI) _____

    G. Systemic vascular resistance (SVR) _____

    H. Pulmonary vascular resistance (PVR) _____

46. What common respiratory problem results in vasoconstriction, or elevated vascular resistance in the pulmonary vessels?

NEUROLOGIC MONITORING

47. Why are the pupils of interest in assessing neurologic status?

48. Name one of the breathing patterns that suggests a neurologic deficit.

49. Describe what happens to the brain for each of the ICP values below.

A. 10 to 15 mm Hg _____

B. 15 to 20 mm Hg _____

C. 30 to 35 mm Hg _____

50. The Glasgow Coma Scale is a popular tool used to assess acute neurologic deficits. What do the following scores mean?

A. 9 to 13 _____

B. < 8 _____

MONITORING RENAL AND LIVER FUNCTION

51. Which two tests are commonly used together to monitor renal function?

52. Define polyuria and oliguria in terms of actual daily output.

53. How is liver function usually evaluated?

NUTRITIONAL MONITORING

54. What does the functional nutritional assessment consist of?

55. What is the most frequently used laboratory measure of nutritional status? What value indicates severe malnutrition?

56. Troubleshooting revolves around which two general problem areas? (See Box 51-14.)

    A. _____

    B. _____

57. Identify common problems and suggest a corrective action.

Clue to Problem	Possible Cause	Corrective Action
Decreased minute ventilation or V_T		
Increased minute ventilation or V_T		
Change in respiratory rate		
Sudden increase in peak airway pressure		
Gradual increase in peak airway pressure		
Sudden decrease in peak airway pressure		
F_IO_2 drift		
Inspired gas temperature too high		
Changes in static pressure		
Changes in ventilator setting		

58. Regardless of the source of the problem, what is always the first priority?

59. If there is any doubt as to the cause or solution of a problem, what action should you take?

WHAT DOES THE NBRC SAY?

Circle the best answer.

60. A 42-year-old patient with a cervical spine injury is being mechanically ventilated in control mode. As you enter the room, the low-pressure alarm is sounding. The patient is connected to the ventilator, but you do not see his chest moving. Your first action would be to _____
    A. manually ventilate the patient with the resuscitation bag
    B. check the alarm settings
    C. observe the exhaled volumes
    D. manually ventilate the patient with the mechanical ventilator

61. After insertion of a Swan-Ganz catheter via the left subclavian vein, a patient's compliance quickly drops. The high-pressure alarm on the ventilator is activated. Breath sounds are absent over the left chest, and the trachea is deviated to the right side. The patient appears extremely anxious. What action should the RCP take?
    A. Use a capnometer to assess ventilation noninvasively.
    B. Recommend administration of Versed.
    C. Call for a portable chest radiograph.
    D. Recommend chest tube insertion.

62. A 38-year-old woman with a diagnosis of myasthenia gravis is being mechanically ventilated. As you enter the room, the high-pressure alarm is sounding. The patient appears anxious. Auscultation reveals coarse bilateral rhonchi. What action should you take at this time?
    A. Manually ventilate the patient.
    B. Check the alarm setting.
    C. Recommend sedation.
    D. Suction the patient.

63. An 89-year-old woman with emphysema is being mechanically ventilated. The high-pressure and high-rate alarms are being activated. Breath sounds are clear. Pulse oximetry and vital sign values are within normal limits. Hemodynamics are normal. ABGs are stable. The patient is very agitated, and her respiratory rate is 32. What are your recommendations?
    A. Administer Versed.
    B. Increase the alarm limit.
    C. Suction the patient.
    D. Call for a portable chest radiograph.

64. The data below are reported for a patient:
    PCWP   25 mm Hg
    PAP   40/24 mm Hg
    CI   1.9 L/min/m^2

    These data suggest which of the following?
    A. Noncardiogenic pulmonary edema
    B. Cardiogenic pulmonary edema
    C. Pulsus paradoxus
    D. Hypovolemia

65. When properly placed, the distal tip of the Swan-Ganz catheter will be located in the _____.
    A. left atrium
    B. right atrium
    C. right ventricle
    D. pulmonary artery

Questions 66 through 68 refer to the following situation:
   A patient is intubated and placed on the ventilator after she develops respiratory failure following hip replacement surgery. The following values are recorded:

    $PaCO_2$ 50 mm Hg
    PaO_2 60 mm Hg
    F_IO_2 0.40
    $PECO_2$ 10 mm Hg
    Tidal volume   800 ml
    Respiratory rate   20

66. These data indicate a dead space–to–tidal volume ratio of _____.
    A. 20%
    B. 40%
    C. 60%
    D. 80%

Chapter **51** **Monitoring the Patient in the Intensive Care Unit**

67. What is the exhaled minute volume?
   A. 8.0 L
   B. 12.0 L
   C. 16.0 L
   D. 20.0 L

68. What is the alveolar minute volume?
   A. 3.2 L
   B. 11.2 L
   C. 12.8 L
   D. 16.0 L

69. The following information is recorded for a patient:

   $\dot{V}O_2$ 200 ml/min
   CaO_2 16 vol %
   CvO_2 12 vol %

   What is the cardiac output?
   A. 2.0 L/min
   B. 3.0 L/min
   C. 4.0 L/min
   D. 5.0 L/min

70. The hemodynamic data below are recorded for a patient who is being mechanically ventilated.

   Cardiac output   3.5 L/min
   PAP   16/8 mm Hg
   PWP   4 mm Hg
   CVP   2 mm Hg
   HR   125/min

   These data probably indicate _____.
   A. hypovolemia
   B. pulmonary hypertension
   C. fluid overload
   D. pulmonary embolism

FOOD FOR THOUGHT

There was an editorial in the journal *Respiratory Care* a few years ago entitled something like this: "The pulmonary artery catheter—it goes in through your arm and you pay through the nose." Think about three questions in relationship to this idea. First, do you think it is important to use top-of-the-line technology in every setting? Second, if your loved one were ill, what would you want for him or her? Third, do you think the average person understands the complexity of "the high cost of medicine"?

52 Discontinuing Ventilatory Support

WORD WIZARD

Please write the meaning of these terms.

ASV _____

MMV _____

PSV _____

PMV _____

RSBI _____

SBT _____

SAT _____

REASONS FOR VENTILATOR DEPENDENCE

1. Define ventilator dependence.

2. What's the difference between weaning from a ventilator and ventilator discontinuation?

    A. Weaning _____

    B. Ventilator discontinuation _____

3. List the five general categories that patients who are being considered for removal from ventilatory support fall into.

    A. _____

    B. _____

    C. _____

    D. _____

    E. _____

4. List four factors that determine total ventilatory workload.

    A. _____

    B. _____

    C. _____

    D. _____

5. Give examples of conditions that adversely affect ventilatory capacity.

   A. CNS drive

     1. _____

     2. _____

     3. _____

     4. _____

   B. Muscle strength

     1. _____

     2. _____

     3. _____

     4. _____

6. Successful discontinuation of ventilatory support is related to which patient's condition?

   A. _____

   B. _____

   C. _____

   D. _____

PATIENT EVALUATION

7. What is the first thing you should evaluate whether you are considering weaning or taking the patient off the ventilator? *The single most important thing.*

8. What are the four questions you should ask?

   A. _____

   B. _____

   C. _____

   D. _____

9. Your board examinations will expect you to identify these classic criteria for weaning from mechanical ventilation. Fill in the criterion values below.

Measurement	Criterion
$PaCO_2$	_____
pH	_____
VC (ml/kg)	_____
Spontaneous V_T	_____
Spontaneous rate	_____
V_E	_____
MVV	_____
MIF (NIF, MIP)	_____
V_D/V_T	_____
$P(A - a)O_2$ on 100%	_____
P/F ratio	_____
PaO_2	_____
Qs/Qt	_____
F_IO_2	_____
f/V_T	_____
Compliance	_____

10. Physical assessment of respiratory muscles may be useful. Describe what you are looking for in this area.

11. Rapid shallow breathing index may be the best overall predictor of weaning outcomes. Calculate the rapid shallow breathing index for a patient who has a spontaneous rate of 25 with a spontaneous volume of 350 ml. What are the criteria for success?

A. Formula _____

B. Calculation _____

C. Criteria _____

12. Give the PaO_2, F_IO_2, and PEEP values that should be met prior to weaning.

A. PaO_2 _____

B. F_IO_2 _____

C. PEEP _____

13. Describe the ways that renal function may affect weaning.

A. Electrolytes _____

B. Fluid balance and urine output _____

C. Metabolic acidosis _____

14. Describe the ideal CNS status needed for discontinuation to be successful.

15. Explain the following indices for weaning:

CROP score: _____

Adverse Factor/Ventilator Score: _____

Weaning index: _____

Burns Weaning Assessment Program: _____

16. What turns out to be the best indices?

17. How can the RT improve conditions in the airway?

18. What environmental considerations should be taken?

WEANING METHODS

19. List the three basic methods of discontinuing ventilatory support.

A. _____

B. _____

C. _____

20. Describe the specific advantage of using the ventilator instead of the T-tube.

21. What is the typical minimum length of time for a spontaneous trial when you are going for rapid discontinuance?

22. What does research show about IMV as it compares to SBTs?

23. From what level of PSV may a patient be extubated?

24. What is an SAT? Why do we do it?

25. When should you repeat the SBT if the patient fails the first trial?

NEWER TECHNIQUES FOR FACILITATING VENTILATOR DISCONTINUANCE

26. Describe mandatory minute ventilation (MMV).

27. Describe adaptive support ventilation (ASV).

28. Why is there a desire to develop a computer-based weaning protocol?

29. When in the weaning process should mobilization of a patient begin?

MONITORING THE PATIENT DURING WEANING

30. What are the two easily monitored and reliable indicators of patient progress during weaning?

A. _____

B. _____

31. What is the simplest way to monitor oxygenation during weaning?

32. Give the expected and excessive changes for each of the following parameters.

Parameter	Expected	Deleterious
Respiratory rate	_____	_____
PaO_2	_____	_____
$PaCO_2$	_____	_____
Heart rate	_____	_____
Blood pressure	_____	_____

EXTUBATION

33. What is the minimum ability required for personnel performing routine extubation?

34. What is the minimum ability required for personnel performing high-risk extubation?

35. What are common patient complaints following extubation?

VENTILATOR DISCONTINUANCE FAILURE

36. Identify five common causes of weaning failure.

A. _____

B. _____

C. _____

D. _____

E. _____

37. What are the alternative care sites for the long-term ventilator patient?

38. Who should be involved in the decision to terminate life support?

39. Discuss the three factors mentioned in your text used to help make the decision.

A 61-year-old woman is placed on the ventilator for respiratory failure for CHF and COPD. Twenty-four hours later, the physician asks for your recommendation regarding weaning. Breath sounds reveal coarse crackles in both bases. Pedal edema is present as well. The following information is obtained.

Spontaneous RR	28
Spontaneous V_t	0.2 L
MIF	-18 cm H_2O
VC	0.6 L
HR	116
BP	90/60
pH	7.33
$PaCO_2$	35 mm Hg
PaO_2	65 (on F_iO_2 0.5)
Cardiac index	2.3

40. What is your assessment of her respiratory status?

41. Has the primary problem been resolved?

42. What is the rapid shallow breathing index?

43. Explain your recommendation regarding initiating weaning. If you recommend weaning, also recommend the method.

A 61-year-old man is placed on the ventilator following open-heart surgery. Twelve hours later, the patient is awake and the physician asks for your recommendation regarding weaning. The following information is obtained:

Spontaneous RR	14
Spontaneous V_T	0.2 L
MIF	−35 cm H_2O
VC	1.2 L
HR	116
BP	90/60
pH	7.37
$PaCO_2$	35 mm Hg
PaO_2	85 (on F_IO_2 0.35)

44. What is your assessment of his respiratory status?

45. Has the primary problem been resolved?

46. What is the rapid shallow breathing index?

47. Explain your recommendation regarding initiating weaning. If you recommend weaning, also recommend a technique.

A 61-year-old man is placed on the ventilator following an acute episode of Guillain-Barré syndrome. At 21 days later, the patient is regaining strength and movement in his limbs. The physician asks for your recommendation regarding weaning. The following information is obtained:

Spontaneous RR	22
Spontaneous V_T	0.22 L
MIF	−20 cm H_2O
VC	1.0 L
HR	116
BP	90/60
pH	7.38
$PaCO_2$	37 mm Hg
PaO_2	70 (on F_IO_2 0.40)

48. What is your assessment of his respiratory status?

49. Has the primary problem been resolved?

50. What is the rapid shallow breathing index?

51. Explain your recommendation regarding initiating weaning. If you recommend weaning, also recommend a technique.

A 5-foot 2-inch, 50-kg, 80-year-old woman has been on the ventilator for 2 days because of hemodynamic instability following open-heart surgery. The vitals are now stable. The physician wants you to conduct a spontaneous breathing trial. You suction the patient and sit her up for trial. Pretrial respiratory rate is 22, MIP is −45 mm Hg, and spontaneous volume is 400 ml. She is placed on a T-piece for 3 minutes with 40% oxygen. After 3 minutes, the f is 25, MIP is −40, and V_T is 420.

52. What would you recommend at this time?

53. What is the RSBI?

54. How long does she need to succeed on the trial before you would consider extubation?

Circle the best answer.

55. Which of the following would you evaluate prior to initiating weaning?
    1. PaO_2
    2. Gag reflex
    3. Spontaneous respiratory rate
    4. Urine output
        A. 1 and 2 only
        B. 1 and 3 only
        C. 2 and 4 only
        D. 3 and 4 only

56. A patient being assessed for readiness for weaning has the following values:

pH	7.36
$PaCO_2$	42 mm Hg
PaO_2	67 mm Hg (F_IO_2 40%)
MIP	-25 cm H_2O
Pulse	105
Respirations	20
VC	12 ml/kg

    What action should the RT recommend at this time?
    A. Initiate a CPAP trial.
    B. Continue with mechanical ventilation.
    C. Initiate breathing exercises to strengthen ventilatory muscles.
    D. Repeat the vital capacity maneuver.

57. Which of the following indicates a readiness to wean?
    A. Spontaneous rate of 28
    B. Spontaneous tidal volume of 200 ml
    C. Negative inspiratory force of 18 cm H_2O
    D. Minute volume of 8 L/min

58. An alert patient is being mechanically ventilated. Settings are:

Mode	SIMV
Rate	2
Tidalvolume (set)	500
F_IO_2	0.30
PEEP	5 cm H_2O

    ABG results 30 minutes after initiating these settings are:

pH	7.37
$PaCO_2$	38 mm Hg
PaO_2	75 mm Hg

    What should the RT recommend at this time?
    A. Increase the set rate to 4.
    B. Discontinue mechanical ventilation.
    C. Decrease the PEEP to 2 cm H_2O.
    D. Decrease the F_IO_2 to 0.21.

59. A patient is being ventilated in the SIMV mode with a rate of 8, volume of 800, and F_IO_2 of 0.40. ABG results show:

pH	7.47
$PaCO_2$	33 mm Hg
PaO_2	88 mm Hg
HCO_3^-	23 mEq/L

What action should the RT recommend in response to these findings?
A. Increase the tidal volume.
B. Increase the F_IO_2.
C. Change to AC mode.
D. Reduce the rate.

60. A patient on SIMV experiences difficulty each time you try to reduce the rate below 6. The patient becomes tachypneic with a rate of 28 and a spontaneous volume of 200. Which of the following modifications would be *least* useful in this situation?
A. Adding pressure support ventilation
B. Transfer back to full ventilatory support
C. Extubation
D. Change to flow triggering

FOOD FOR THOUGHT

61. What is the single best approach to weaning?

53 Neonatal and Pediatric Respiratory Care

WORD WIZARD

Write out the words for these acronyms.

AGA _____

CPAP _____

ECMO _____

HFV _____

INO _____

PPHN _____

PDA _____

ROP _____

FETAL ASSESSMENT

1. Assessment of the newborn begins with maternal history. Identify three conditions that are likely to result in a baby who is small for its gestational age.

   A. _____

   B. _____

   C. _____

2. Identify five maternal factors likely to lead to premature delivery.

   A. _____

   B. _____

   C. _____

   D. _____

   E. _____

3. What maternal metabolic condition is likely to result in an infant who is large for its gestational age?

4. Briefly describe each of the following tests.
   A. Ultrasonography

   B. Amniocentesis (Be sure to include LS ratio and PG. Also, include normal and abnormal values and what the terms mean.)

   C. Fetal heart rate monitoring (Be sure to discuss accelerations, decelerations, and heart rate values and what they mean.)

   D. Fetal blood gas analysis (Include normal values and describe the relationship between fetal scalp gases and arterial blood gases.)

NEWBORN ASSESSMENT

5. When are Apgar scores taken?

6. Fill in the chart regarding the Apgar scoring system.

	SIGN	0	1	2
A.	Heart rate			
B.	Respiration			
C.	Muscle tone			
D.	Reflex			
E.	Color			

Chapter 53 Neonatal and Pediatric Respiratory Care

7. What term is used to describe the following weeks of gestation?

    A. Before 38 weeks _____

    B. 38 to 42 weeks _____

    C. After 42 weeks _____

8. Name the two common systems used for assessing gestational age based on physical characteristics and neurologic signs.

    A. _____

    B. _____

9. Explain the abbreviations and identify the weights that correspond to the following terms.

	ABBREVIATION	FULL NAME	WEIGHTS/PERCENTS
A.	VLBW		
B.	LBW		
C.	AGA		
D.	LGA		
E.	SGA		

ASSESSING THE NEWBORN

10. State the normal range for a full-term infant's vital signs.

    A. Heart rate _____

    B. Respiratory rate _____

    C. Blood pressure _____

11. Explain the significance of each sign.

    A. Nasal flaring _____

    B. Cyanosis _____

    C. Expiratory grunting _____

    D. Retractions _____

    E. Paradoxical breathing _____

12. What scoring system is used to grade the severity of underlying lung disease?

13. How is the need for surfactant determined?

14. What are the two usual sites for obtaining blood gas samples in infants?

   A. _____

   B. _____

15. List the ABG values for preterm and term infants at birth.

	PARAMETER	PRETERM (1 TO 5 HOURS)	NORMAL TERM (5 HOURS)	NORMAL PRETERM INFANTS (5 DAYS)
A.	pH			
B.	$PaCO_2$			
C.	PaO_2			

RESPIRATORY CARE TECHNIQUES

16. Considering its hazards, we need to agree on the safe limits for oxygen therapy. Give the accepted ranges for these parameters.

   A. F_iO_2 < _____ %

   B. Preemie SpO_2 _____ to _____

17. How could oxygen cause heart problems to worsen in some newborns?

18. Compare the use of the following oxygen delivery devices.

	DEVICE	AGE	ADVANTAGE	DISADVANTAGE
A.	AEM			
B.	Cannula			
C.	Incubator			
D.	Hood			
E.	Tent			

19. Name four conditions in which secretion retention is common in children.

   A. _____

   B. _____

   C. _____

   D. _____

20. Why is it so important to monitor ALL aspects of infants who need bronchial hygiene therapy?

21. What type of device is used for patients who are intubated?

22. In terms of humidification, what's important about volume and water level for babies on ventilators?

23. What factors could affect the delivery of humidity from a servo-controlled heated humidifier to an infant who is mechanically ventilated?

24. State the four methods you can use to deliver aerosol medications to children.

A. _____

B. _____

C. _____

D. _____

AIRWAY MANAGEMENT

25. Identify the correct ET size and suction catheter size for these children.

	AGE/WEIGHT	ET INTERNAL DIAMETER (ID)	LENGTH (ORAL)	SUCTION
A.	< 1000 g			
B.	1000 to 2000 g			
C.	2000 to 3000 g			
D.	> 3000 g			
E.	2 years			
F.	6 years			

26. State the two formulas for calculating tube diameter.

27. What is the consequence of placing an ET tube that is too small in an infant?

28. Estimate the correct tube size for a 4-year-old using the first formula in question 26.

29. Which laryngoscope blade is usually used for infant intubation?

30. Which airway can be used as an alternative to intubation in children?

31. What are the recommended vacuum pressures for suctioning infants and children?

    A. Infants _____

    B. Children _____

32. Identify the criteria for initiating chest compressions after delivery.

CONTINUOUS POSITIVE AIRWAY PRESSURE

33. What is the specific indication for CPAP? Give the blood gas values.

    A. Indication _____

    B. Blood gas values _____

34. Discuss adjustment of CPAP in infants.
    A. Start at:

    B. Adjust in increments of:

HIGH-FLOW NASAL CANNULA

35. What is the range of flow given for the new cannulas?

36. What problem may occur if the prongs on a high-flow system fit tightly in the nares?

MECHANICAL VENTILATION

37. What pulmonary diseases typically require mechanical ventilation?

    A. _____

    B. _____

    C. _____

    D. _____

38. Give the range of PIP for infants for initiating time-cycled, pressure-limited ventilation.

39. Identify the inspiratory time ranges that should be set for these age groups.

    A. Neonates _____

    B. Older children _____

40. What PEEP levels are usually used in neonates for initiating ventilation?

41. What range of volumes is normally used when volume ventilation is selected?

42. Why would it be common to observe lower exhaled than inhaled volumes in pediatric patients?

43. List five considerations made prior to extubation.

    A. _____

    B. _____

    C. _____

    D. _____

    E. _____

HIGH FREQUENCY VENTILATION

44. Identify the two common characteristics of HFV.

    A. V_T _____

    B. Rate _____

45. What are the three types of HFV? Which is most common?

    A. _____

    B. _____

    C. _____

    Most common? _____

46. How would you wean a patient from HFV?

SPECIALTY GASES

47. What effect does INO have on oxygenation?

48. Two big problems exist with NO inhalation. Explain.
    A. Rebound pulmonary hypertension

    B. Altered hemoglobin

49. Why is heliox typically used? When is it less effective?

Circle the best answer.

50. Which of the following tests would be useful in determining lung maturity?
    A. Sweat chloride
    B. L/S ratio
    C. Fetal hemoglobin
    D. Pneumogram

51. Calculate the Apgar score for a crying infant who has a heart rate of 120, actively moves, and sneezes when a catheter is put in the nose but has blue extremities.
    A. 5
    B. 6
    C. 7
    D. 9

52. The simplest way to apply CPAP to treat hypoxemia in an infant is to use _____
    A. nasal prongs
    B. nasal mask
    C. full-face mask
    D. oxygen hood

53. Excessive oxygen delivery to newborns may raise the risk of
    A. pneumonia.
    B. retinopathy of prematurity.
    C. cystic fibrosis.
    D. PPHN.

54. What vacuum pressure would you set for suctioning a newborn?
    A. 40-60 mm Hg
    B. 60-80 mm Hg
    C. 80-100 mm Hg
    D. 80-120 mm Hg

55. What size endotracheal tube would you recommend for a 1500-g preemie?
    A. 2.5
    B. 3.0
    C. 3.5
    D. 4.0

FOOD FOR THOUGHT

If you choose to work in this field, it would be a good idea to take the Neonatal/Pediatric Specialist Examination to test your knowledge and demonstrate your competence in this specialty area.

54 Patient Education and Health Promotion

WORD WIZARD

Write out the definition for each of these terms.

1. Affective domain _____

2. Cognitive domain _____

3. Health education _____

4. Health promotion _____

5. Psychomotor domain _____

PATIENT EDUCATION

6. List the top three causes of death in the United States.

   1. _____

   2. _____

   3. _____

7. Why is educating the public about these illnesses so important?

8. Why should the development of written objectives for patient teaching be considered?

9. How can the RT state an objective in measurable terms during patient education sessions?

   A. Begin with a _____

   B. Write an action _____

   C. Add a condition _____

   D. Write a standard _____

10. Give an example of an objective for each of the following learning domains.

	DOMAIN	OBJECTIVE
A.	Cognitive	
B.	Affective	
C.	Psychomotor	

389

11. Which of the learning domains should be evaluated before you proceed with patient education?

12. What is the key to motivating patients to learn?

13. What is the key to teaching psychomotor skills? How can you confirm that a patient or family member has learned a new skill?

14. Give an example from the text of how to relate psychomotor skills a patient uses every day to help make the transition from everyday life to therapy.

Teaching Children as Compared With Teaching Adults

15. How is teaching children different from teaching adults? How is it the same?

16. Where could you find resource materials to help in teaching children with asthma?

17. What suggestions are given for rewarding performance?

Evaluation

18. What process answers the question "Has the patient learned?" When should you begin to develop this process?

19. Describe some of the formal and informal ways you can tell if a patient has met affective domain objectives.

20. What is the primary goal of health education?

21. Learning activities must incorporate values and beliefs of the learner. List four factors that need to be considered in this area.

    A. _____

    B. _____

    C. _____

    D. _____

22. How do the personal characteristics of the educator impact learning?

HEALTH PROMOTION AND DISEASE PREVENTION

23. Compare the standard medical approach to health in the United States with the public health model.

24. What are two broad goals of the Healthy People 2020 initiative?

25. Discuss how RTs might participate in the management of COPD through education.

26. Besides the hospital, name four other settings where RTs would be likely to function as individual counselors or public health advocates.

A. _____

B. _____

C. _____

D. _____

CASE STUDY

Your text has several good cases in the form of "Mini-Clinis," so let's do something else. Suppose you had to teach your classmates how to use a peak flowmeter. Write three objectives for this topic for each domain using behavioral terms.

27. Cognitive domain
   A.

   B.

   C.

28. Affective domain
   A.

   B.

   C.

29. Psychomotor domain

   A.

   B.

   C.

30. How long would your teaching session last?

31. Give examples of how you would involve the following senses in your session.

   A. Hearing _____

   B. Seeing _____

   C. Touching _____

   D. Writing _____

   E. Speaking _____

32. Give an example of how you would measure learning for each domain.

   A. Cognitive _____

   B. Affective _____

   C. Psychomotor _____

WHAT DOES THE NBRC SAY?

33. The best way to ensure that a patient has learned to properly administer a bronchodilator via MDI is to
   A. ask the patient to answer questions regarding inhaler use.
   B. give the patient appropriate literature regarding MDI use.
   C. ask the patient to demonstrate how to use the inhaler.
   D. have the patient explain when he is to use the MDI.

34. Why do you think the public should be educated about the risk factors for the top causes of death?

35. How is teaching other caregivers different from teaching patients or family members?

55 Cardiopulmonary Rehabilitation

WORD WIZARD

Match the following terms and acronyms to their definitions.

Terms and Acronyms	Definitions
1. _____ ADL	A. Physical activities designed to strengthen muscles and improve O_2 utilization.
2. _____ Borg scale	B. Measure of an individual's ability to perform common tasks.
3. _____ CORF	C. Point where there is insufficient O_2 to meet the demands of energy metabolism.
4. _____ Karvonen's formula	D. Measure of an individual's perception of breathing difficulty.
5. _____ Progressive resistance	E. Cardiac goal for aerobic conditioning based on 65% of maximum O_2 consumption.
6. _____ OBLA	F. Ratio of CO_2 production to O_2 consumption.
7. _____ Reconditioning	G. Medicare-approved facility that provides ambulatory rehabilitation services.
8. _____ Respiratory quotient	H. Common method used to calculate target heart rate for exercise.
9. _____ Target heart rate	I. Training method that gradually increases muscle workloads.

DEFINITIONS AND GOALS

10. What event placed a focus on hospital readmissions and the importance of pulmonary rehabilitation?

11. In your own words, define pulmonary rehabilitation.

12. List three general goals of pulmonary rehabilitation.

A. _____

B. _____

C. _____

13. How do clinical and social sciences play a role in establishing ways to improve the patient's quality of life?

14. Define OBLA and describe it in relation to physical reconditioning.

15. How can you estimate MVV using simple spirometry?

16. Identify the three general ways that reconditioning will increase exercise tolerance.
    A. _____
    B. _____
    C. _____

17. Compare the roles of psychosocial and physical methods in terms of outcomes of rehabilitation.

18. Describe the two-way relationship of physical reconditioning and psychosocial support.

STRUCTURE OF A PULMONARY REHABILITATION PROGRAM

19. Why is it so important to have specific objectives for the program goals? How should these objectives be stated?
    A.

    B.

20. List five accepted benefits of exercise reconditioning.

    A. _____

    B. _____

    C. _____

    D. _____

    E. _____

21. Research literature clearly shows that rehabilitation has proven benefits. What is the effect of rehabilitation on the progression of the disease?

22. Name three common goals (*not objectives*) for rehabilitation programs.

    A. _____

    B. _____

    C. _____

23. Who manages the overall care in a program and screens the prospective patients?

24. What is the first step in patient evaluation for a pulmonary rehab program?

25. List four tests that should be included with the physical examination.

    A. _____

    B. _____

    C. _____

    D. _____

26. Two tests are typically conducted to assess cardiopulmonary status. State two purposes for these tests.
    A. Exercise evaluation

        1. _____

        2. _____

    B. Pulmonary function testing

        1. _____

        2. _____

27. List two contraindications to exercise testing.

    A. _____

    B. _____

28. Identify four physiologic parameters that should be monitored during exercise testing.

A. _____

B. _____

C. _____

D. _____

29. List four general groups of patients included in pulmonary rehabilitation programs.

A. _____

B. _____

C. _____

D. _____

30. What are the benefits of grouping patients together on the basis of severity and overall ability?

31. Give one benefit and one drawback of the open-ended program model.

A. Benefit: _____

B. Drawback: _____

32. Give one benefit and one drawback to the traditional closed design.

A. Benefit: _____

B. Drawback: _____

33. Describe Medicare coverage for pulmonary rehabilitation.

34. Describe two ways to set target heart rate for patient exercise.

A. Formula _____

B. Estimate _____

35. Describe a typical walking exercise program. What is our minimum walk time?

36. What is the basic concept behind ventilatory muscle training?

37. Briefly discuss the following high-priority program educational components.
   A. Breathing control

   B. Stress management

   C. Medications

   D. Diet

38. What is the ideal class size for a rehabilitation program? What external factor affects this ideal?

39. Give specific examples for each of the following sources of program reimbursement.
   A. Nongovernment health insurance _____
   B. Federal and state health insurance _____
   C. Ancillary insurance _____
   D. Other options _____

40. What is/are the most likely cause(s) of lack of measurable improvement within a pulmonary rehabilitation program?

41. Potential hazards do exist in pulmonary rehabilitation. Give one from each category:

A. Cardio _____

B. Blood gas _____

C. Muscular _____

D. Miscellaneous _____

CASE STUDIES

Case 1

An alert 55-year-old man with long-standing asthma and COPD is admitted for acute exacerbation of his illness following a "chest cold." This is the fourth admission for this patient in the past 3 months. He tells you that he has had to quit his job and take early retirement because of his lung problems.

42. What concerns does this situation raise?

43. Explain the benefits of entering a rehabilitation program to this patient.

Case 2

A 57-year-old woman with chronic bronchitis is enrolled in your pulmonary rehabilitation program. During walking exercises, she complains of dyspnea and will not continue with the walk.

44. What assessments would be useful in this situation?

45. Give several possible methods for modifying the exercise program to improve this patient's compliance.

WHAT DOES THE NBRC SAY?

Circle the answers.

46. A COPD patient has enrolled in a pulmonary rehabilitation program. The patient should be informed that the program will help provide all of the benefits *except* _____.
    A. increased physical endurance
    B. improved PFT results
    C. increased activity levels
    D. improved cardiovascular function

47. During an exercise test a patient is able to reach a maximum heart rate of 120. His resting heart rate is 70. What target heart rate would you recommend for this patient during aerobic conditioning?
    A. 70 beats per minute
    B. 85 beats per minute
    C. 100 beats per minute
    D. 115 beats per minute

48. Which of the following tests would be useful in assessing ventilatory reserve during exercise testing?
    A. Forced vital capacity
    B. Maximum voluntary ventilation
    C. Body plethysmography
    D. Single breath nitrogen washout

FOOD FOR THOUGHT

All throughout *Egan's* we find references to the Borg scale. This scale is a valuable tool that can be easily used at the bedside or in the rehabilitation setting.

49. Describe the Borg scale. What is the value of this instrument?

50. Compare and contrast cardiac rehabilitation with pulmonary rehabilitation.

56 Respiratory Care in Alternative Settings

WORD WIZARD

Write out the meanings of the following acronyms.

1. CMS _____

2. DME _____

3. NIV _____

4. LTACH _____

5. SNF _____

6. TTOT _____

MORE RECENT DEVELOPMENTS AND TRENDS

7. What is the most common alternative site for health care?

8. How has the Patient Protection and Affordable Care Act (ACA) of 2010 affected alternative settings?

RELEVANT TERMS AND GOALS

9. List five areas of nonacute or alternative care.

A. _____

B. _____

C. _____

D. _____

E. _____

10. Describe the LTACH and its relationship to respiratory care.

11. What is subacute care?

12. List four common respiratory care services provided in alternative settings.

    A. _____

    B. _____

    C. _____

    D. _____

13. List three of the benefits of respiratory home care.

    A. _____

    B. _____

    C. _____

    Now list three typical disease states that need our help.

    D. _____

    E. _____

    F. _____

STANDARDS

14. What is the purpose of the Medicare Provider Certification Program?

15. Who is responsible for accreditation of companies that provide home care services?

16. What do RTs like about working in alternative care settings?

17. Compare traditional and alternative settings in terms of the following areas.

AREA	TRADITIONAL	ALTERNATIVE
A. Diagnostic tests		
B. Equipment		
C. Supervision		
D. Patient assessment		
E. Work schedule		
F. Time constraints		

DISCHARGE PLANNING

18. Explain the role of the following practitioners in the alternative care setting team.

A. Utilization and review _____

B. Social services _____

C. Physical therapy _____

D. Psychiatrist _____

E. DME supplier _____

19. How can you confirm that a nonprofessional caregiver is able to perform care?

20. Discuss items in the home environment that must be assessed prior to discharge.
A. Accessibility

B. Equipment

C. Environment

OXYGEN THERAPY

21. Why do so many people use oxygen in alternative care settings in the United States?

22. State two of the documented benefits of long-term oxygen therapy.

A. _____

B. _____

23. Describe the six elements that must be included in a home oxygen prescription.

A. _____

B. _____

C. _____

D. _____

E. _____

F. _____

24. The AARC Clinical Practice Guidelines for Oxygen in the Home clearly state the indications for oxygen outside the acute care hospital.

A. Adults, etc., > 28 days PaO_2 ≤ _____ mm Hg, or SaO_2 ≤ _____.

B. Cor pulmonale, CHF, or critical > 56% PaO_2 ≤ _____ or SaO_2 ≤ _____.

C. Ambulation, sleep, or exercise if SaO_2 falls below _____%.

25. What are the two primary uses of compressed oxygen cylinders in alternative settings?

A. E cylinder _____

B. H cylinder (or M) _____

26. How do flowmeters used in alternative settings differ from those used in the hospital?

27. What is the typical range of oxygen percentage a concentrator will supply?

A. 1 to 2 L/min _____

B. > 5 L/min _____

28. What effect will the concentrator have on a patient's electrical bill?

29. Describe some of the methods for avoiding communication problems with patients receiving home oxygen therapy.

30. List at least four areas that should be evaluated when checking a home patient's oxygen concentrator.

A. _____

B. _____

C. _____

D. _____

31. When a patient is placed on an oxygen-conserving device, how would you determine the correct liter flow to use?

32. What actions should a patient who is wearing transtracheal oxygen take if he believes the catheter isn't working properly?

33. State the three main problems associated with insertion of the transtracheal catheter (see Box 51-4).

A. _____

B. _____

C. _____

34. Describe the basic methods for avoiding complications of transtracheal catheters.

VENTILATORY SUPPORT IN ALTERNATIVE SETTINGS

35. Give examples for each of the three main groups of patients who are placed on ventilators in the alternative care setting.

A. Nocturnal ventilation

1. _____

2. _____

3. _____

B. Continuous mechanical ventilation

1. _____

2. _____

3. _____

C. Terminally ill

1. _____

2. _____

36. Invasive long-term ventilation is always provided via what type of airway?

37. Describe the emergency situations a family must be able to deal with in caring for a home ventilator patient.

38. What options exist for patients who do not want invasive ventilation and cannot use NIV?

39. What options are available on invasive positive pressure ventilator systems during power failures or if a patient wishes to be mobile?

40. What is the biggest challenge associated with NIV?

OTHER MODES OF POSTACUTE VENTILATION IN ALTERNATIVE SITES

41. What is the primary use of bland aerosols in the alternative care setting?

42. What is the major problem with delivery of bland aerosols?

43. What is the most common clinical problem with the CPAP apparatus?

44. Discuss solutions to the common complaint of nasal dryness.

45. Apnea monitors alert parents or caregivers of what serious signs? How long do they need the monitor?
   A. Condition _____
   B. Duration of monitoring _____

46. Describe the main areas you would check during initial screening of a patient following admission to an alternative care facility.

47. What areas would be important to assess besides the usual vital signs and evaluation of the respiratory system?

48. How often should a member of the home care team perform a follow-up evaluation for patients receiving respiratory care treatments? What factors should be considered in determining the frequency of visits?

EQUIPMENT DISINFECTION AND MAINTENANCE

49. Describe the process for cleaning a home nebulizer (for example):

A. _____

B. _____

C. _____

50. Describe the guidelines for using water in humidifiers and nebulizers.

51. What is the most important principle of infection control in the home setting?

PALLIATIVE CARE

52. According to the World Health Organization, palliative care involves control of what two debilitating symptoms?

A. _____

B. _____

53. What is hospice?

Case 1

A 70-year-old with COPD is discharged with an order for home oxygen. The room air blood gas prior to discharge is:

pH   7.47
$PaCO_2$ 33 mm Hg
PaO_2 62 mm Hg
SaO_2 92%

Medicare returns the CMN as "disapproved" on the basis that this patient does not meet the PO_2 saturation criteria for home oxygen.

54. Make an argument for keeping the patient on oxygen based on your knowledge of respiratory physiology. You won't find a clear answer in the text.

Case 2

A home care patient whom you are seeing uses an oxygen concentrator. He calls you to say that he doesn't think he is getting an adequate amount of flow from his cannula.

55. What are some possible causes of this problem?

56. What would you suggest the patient do to quickly check the cannula?

Case 3

An active 49-year-old with α_1-antitrypsin deficiency is to be discharged with home oxygen. The prescription is for 2 L/min continuous oxygen.

57. What system would you recommend for this patient to use at home?

58. What about a portable system?

Circle the answer.

59. A patient with a tracheostomy is to receive humidification via a nebulizer in his home. With regard to water for the nebulizer, which of the following would be the most appropriate choice for the home setting?
    1. Sterile distilled water should be obtained from the DME provider.
    2. Tap water is sufficient for the home setting if the nebulizer is cleaned properly.
    3. Bottled water can be used as long as it is distilled.
    4. Tap water that is boiled may be used for up to 24 hours.
        A. 1 and 3 only
        B. 1 and 4 only
        C. 2 and 3 only
        D. 2 and 4 only

60. Which of the following actions would an RT perform during the monthly check of a home oxygen concentrator system?
    1. Replacement of the silica pellets in the sieve bed
    2. Analysis of the F_IO_2 delivered by the concentrator
    3. Filter replacement
    4. Evaluation of the concentrator's electrical system
        A. 1 and 2 only
        B. 2 and 3 only
        C. 1 and 4 only
        D. 3 and 4 only

61. A patient who is using oxygen at home occasionally needs to go out for health care appointments. What type of portable system would you recommend for this patient?
    A. E cylinder with standard flowmeter.
    B. E cylinder with conserving device.
    C. Small liquid oxygen reservoir.
    D. Patients can go out for short periods without supplemental oxygen.

62. A respiratory care practitioner determines that a cuirass-type negative pressure ventilator is now reading a pressure of −20 cm H_2O, when it should be cycling at −35 cm H_2O. The patient is in no distress, but the measured tidal volume is 200 ml lower than the desired volume. The practitioner should _____.
    A. begin manual ventilation of the patient
    B. check for leaks in the system
    C. increase the vacuum setting
    D. increase the amount of air in the cuff

Think about the care you would want for your mother, father, or even yourself. Wouldn't it be wonderful to be able to care for your loved one (or yourself) safely in a serene environment of an alternative care setting versus a loud, busy, hospital?